中英对照图文版
In both Chinese and English

针灸史话

Historical
Narratives
of Acupuncture
and Moxibustion

主　编　张立剑
Editor in Chief　ZHANG Li-jian

副主编　申玮红
Associate Editor in Chief　SHEN Wei-hong

主　译　刘俊岭
Translator in Chief　LIU Jun-ling

英文翻译　洪　涛　余　敏
申玮红
Translators　HONG Tao, YU Min, SHEN Wei-hong

第2版　2nd Edition

人民卫生出版社

图书在版编目（CIP）数据

针灸史话：中英对照图文版 / 张立剑主编 . —2 版
. —北京：人民卫生出版社，2020
ISBN 978-7-117-29308-2

Ⅰ.①针… Ⅱ.①张… Ⅲ.①针灸学-医学史-中国
-汉、英 Ⅳ.①R245-092

中国版本图书馆 CIP 数据核字（2019）第 284061 号

| 人卫智网 | www.ipmph.com | 医学教育、学术、考试、健康， |
| | | 购书智慧智能综合服务平台 |
| 人卫官网 | www.pmph.com | 人卫官方资讯发布平台 |

针灸史话（中英对照图文版）
第 2 版

主　　编：张立剑
出版发行：人民卫生出版社（中继线 010-59780011）
地　　址：北京市朝阳区潘家园南里 19 号
邮　　编：100021
E - mail：pmph @ pmph.com
购书热线：010-59787592　010-59787584　010-65264830
印　　刷：北京顶佳世纪印刷有限公司
经　　销：新华书店
开　　本：787 × 1092　1/16　印张：13
字　　数：276 千字
版　　次：2010 年 4 月第 1 版　2020 年 3 月第 2 版
　　　　　2020 年 3 月第 2 版第 1 次印刷（总第 2 次印刷）
标准书号：ISBN 978-7-117-29308-2
定　　价：150.00 元

打击盗版举报电话：010-59787491　E-mail：WQ @ pmph.com
质量问题联系电话：010-59787234　E-mail：zhiliang @ pmph.com

# 主编简介
## About the Author

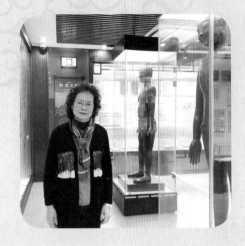

**张立剑**，从事针灸文献与信息化研究工作，正高级职称。主持或参与省部级、国家级科研课题 10 余项，获省部级奖 7 项。主编《朱琏与针灸》《中医针灸》《针灸史话》《针灸图说》（2012 年首届全国优秀中医药文化科普图书）等，在核心期刊发表相关学术论文 30 篇。

Ms. ZHANG Li-jian, professor, has been devoting herself to the research of literature and informatization of acupuncture and moxibustion. By now, Prof. ZHANG has taken charge of or taken part in over 10 scientific and technological projects at provincial, ministerial and national levels, and has got 7 provincial and ministerial awards.

Her publications include *ZHU Lian and Acupuncture-Moxibustion*, *Acupuncture and Moxibustion of Traditional Chinese Medicine*, *Historical Narratives of Acupuncture and Moxibustion*, *Illustration of Acupuncture and Moxibustion* (1st National Outstanding Publications in 2012 of Traditional Chinese Medicine Popular Science Books), etc. Moreover, she also has 30 academic articles published on Chinese core academic journals.

# 内容简介
## Introduction

2010 年 11 月"中医针灸"入选"人类非物质文化遗产代表名录",国内外越来越多的人渴望学习针灸,了解针灸发展的历史源流,为此,我们再版《针灸史话》一书。此次再版,对某些专题进行了精编删减,同时,增加了数个具有重要历史意义的专题,并对上版中的若干专题进行了重新研究、考证和再归纳,使全书更能准确地反映针灸的历史全貌,更具权威与价值。

本书图文并茂,中英对照,集 220 帧图片、列 84 个专题,按针灸发展的历史主线形象地呈现了针灸数千年发展的概貌。

Ever since acupuncture and moxibustion of traditional Chinese medicine (TCM) was inscribed on the list of "Intangible Cultural Heritage of Humanity" in November 2010, many people at home and abroad are eager to learn acupuncture and moxibustion therapies and want to know its origin and historical development. In order to meet the demand, we anew revised the book *Historical Narratives of Acupuncture and Moxibustion* by deleting several topics and supplementing some special subjects involving important historical events after careful re-investigation, re-examination and further refinement, making the whole book fully reflect historical profile and possess more authoritative and valuable basic knowledge for the public.

This book, composed of 220 pictures and 84 special topics, written in both Chinese and English, provides vivid insights into the outline of the development of acupuncture and moxibustion in the past thousands of years.

# 目 录
## Contents

# 1

# 伏羲、黄帝与针砭
Fuxi and Huangdi (Yellow Emperor) and stone-needle

　　传说中的伏羲与黄帝是针砭的发明者。西晋著名文学家、医学家皇甫谧所著的《帝王世纪》认为，作八卦、教人渔猎的伏羲曾"尝百草而制九针"。以保存大量古代传说而著称的宋代的《路史》中亦载伏羲"尝草治砭，以制民疾"。同样是西晋皇甫谧所著的我国现存第一部针灸学专著《针灸甲乙经》序中有言："黄帝咨访岐伯、伯高、少俞之徒，……而针道生焉。"唐代孙思邈所著《备急千金要方》序中亦载："黄帝受命，创制九针。"

　　其实，针砭的发明究竟归属于哪位传说人物并不十分重要，至少这种有关其起源的追溯表明了其历史相当久远。

Chinese lengendary Fuxi and Huangdi (Yellow Emperor) are the inventors of stone-needle. HUANGFU Mi, a well-known writer and medical specialist from the Western Jin Dynasty pointed out in his book *Diwang Shiji* (《帝王世纪》*Chronological Records of Emperors and Kings*) that Fuxi, a legendary founder of Chinese polity, created Eight Trigrams and taught people to fish and hunt, once "tasted hundreds of herbs and made nine types of needles". In book *Lushi* (《路史》*History of Roads*) of the Song Dynasty which is well-known for preserving a lot of ancient legends, there is also a record that Fuxi "tasted medicinal herbs and made stone needles for the treatment of civilian's ills". It could be also found in the preface of HUANGFU Mi's another book *Zhenjiu Jiayi Jing*, the extant first monograph on acupuncture and moxibustion in China, that "Huangdi consulted Qibo, Bogao, Shaoyu et al, ... then, made the acupuncture treatment approaches clear". SUN Si-miao from the Tang Dynasty wrote in his book *Beiji Qianjin Yaofang* that "Huangdi was ordered to create nine types of needles".

In fact, it's not important that which legendary personage created stone-needle. What is important is that its application may be traced back to the remote historical period in ancient China.

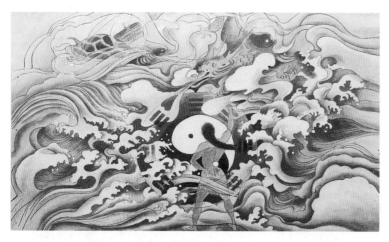

◇伏羲制八卦图

　摄于湖南中医药大学针灸陈列馆

Fuxi created Eight Trigrams
Photographed in the Museum of Acupuncture and Moxibustion of Hunan University of TCM

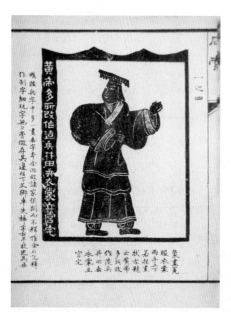

◇汉画像石黄帝像摹本

　引自《针灸史图录》（王雪苔主编，中国医药科技出版社，1987年）

A copy of the Han Dynasty's Stone portrait of Huangdi
Cited from book *Zhenjiushi Tulu* (《针灸史图录》*Picturial Records of History of Acupuncture and Moxibustion*) (Editor-in-chief WANG Xue-tai, published by China Medical Science and Technology Press in 1987)

##  伏羲与黄帝

伏羲是中华民族人文始祖。相传伏羲人首蛇身,与其妹女娲成婚,生儿育女,成为人类的始祖。同时,伏羲还创造了中华民族的一些古老文化。他根据天地间阴阳变化之理,创制八卦,即以八种形状简明却寓意深刻的符号来概括、描述天地之间的事物。相传他也开创了中华医药的悠久文明,为民族的繁衍生息做出了重要贡献。

黄帝为传说中远古时代华夏民族的共主、五帝之首,相传其姓公孙,出生于轩辕之丘,故名号轩辕(天鼋)氏,在姬水生长成人,所以又以姬为姓,后来在有熊建立国家,故亦称有熊氏。关于黄帝的传说中最令人耳熟能详的要数他与炎帝、蚩尤的战争了,最终黄帝取得了胜利,被各部落拥戴为部落联盟领袖。黄帝时期,已发明养蚕、舟车、文字、音律、医学、算数等,并得到发展,他的功劳为后世所称赞,被誉为华夏的"人文初祖"。

## *Fuxi and Huangdi*

Fuxi was the first ancestor of the Chinese nation. According to legend, Fuxi with human head and snake body was married to her sister Nuwa, they gave birth to children and became the first ancestor of mankind. At the same time, Fuxi created ancient Chinese culture. Based on the changes of yin-yang between the heaven and earth, he developed the Eight Trigrams to sum up and describe phenomena in nature by eight simple symbols with profound implications. It was said that he also created a long-standing civilization of Chinese medicine, and made important contributions to the growth and prosperity of the Chinese nation.

Huangdi, the Yellow Emperor, was the head of the Five Emperors of the common ancestors of Huaxia nationality in the period of remote antiquity of ancient China. His original surname was Gongsun, and he was born in the hill of Xuanyuan, so his given name was Xuanyuan (Tianyuan) family. Since he grew up in Jishui, he had another surname of Ji. Later he established a country in Youxiong, so he was also called Youxiong. The most famous story about Huangdi is that he fought with Yandi and Chiyou, and eventually he won the victory and was respected as the leader of the tribal alliance. During the Yellow Emperor period, silkworm rearing, boating, writing, music, medicine, arithmetic were invented and developed. His contributions were appreciated by later generations, and he was known as the "first ancestor of humanities" in China.

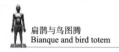

# 2

# 扁鹊与鸟图腾
Bianque and bird totem

　　相传神鸟"扁鹊"与针砭起源也有着密切关系。20世纪70年代,山东微山两城山出土有东汉画像石"扁鹊行医针砭图",图中生动刻画一"半人半鹊"之神鸟以针砭等工具给人治病,其旁阴刻有"山鹊"字样。此神鸟当为上古时期之扁鹊,反映了古代东夷地区原始的鸟图腾崇拜(古有"鸟夷羽民"之说,古人以鸟为图腾,认为鸟具有某种神力,如鸟能交通人神,羽化升仙,祛疾增寿等),揭示了东夷针砭之术的起源。

　　后来,"扁鹊"一词成为对后世名医的尊称,尤其是战国时期的秦越人,直接被以"扁鹊"称之。

It is said that the mythical bird "Bianque" is closely related to the origin of "Zhen Bian" (stone-needle). In 1970s, a stone relief carving, named as "Bianque performing stone-needle picture" from the Eastern Han Dynasty period, was unearthed in Liangchengshan of Weishan County of Shandong Province. The stone relief is engraved with a vivid "half-human magpie" (human head and bird body) treating a patient using a stone needle and with an incised word "山鹊 (mountain magpie)" nearby. This half-human magpie is speculated to be "Bianque" in the antediluvian period of China, reflecting the primitive bird totem worship custom in the ancient coastal region of Bohai Bay (where a saying about "Niaoyi Yumin" existed in the ancient times, i.e., the indigenous people believed that the bird is a totem and has a sort of extraordinary power, for instance, being able in communicating the human to gods, becoming celestial being, and helping the patient remove pathogens to prolong life span, etc.). All of these possibly reveal the origin of stone needling technique in the coastal area of Bohai Bay in ancient China.

Later on, the word "Bianque" gradually becomes an honorific title for well-known physicians, like QIN Yue-ren in the Warring States period.

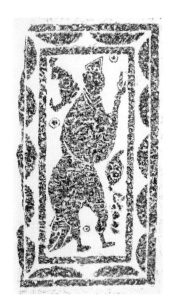

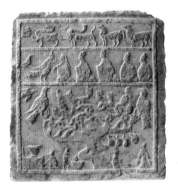

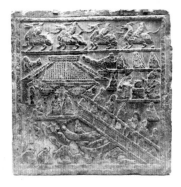

◇东汉画像石扁鹊拓片
　山东省济南市博物馆藏

Bianque rubbings of stone relief from
the Eastern Han Dynasty
Preserved by the Museum of Jinan
City, Shandong Province

◇东汉画像石扁鹊砭刺图
　山东省曲阜市孔庙藏

Eastern Han Dynasty stone relief with
Bianque's stone-needle performing
Preserved by Confucius Temple of
Qufu City, Shandong Province

◇东汉画像石扁鹊针刺图
　中国国家博物馆藏

Eastern Han Dynasty stone relief with
Bianque's acupuncture needle performing
Preserved by National Museum of China

 鸟图腾与医学

　　古人以鸟为图腾，鸟能祛疾安泰，助人长寿，引人升仙，东晋葛洪《抱朴子》中载"千岁之鸟，万岁之禽，皆人面而鸟身，寿亦如其名"，因而赋予它健康长寿繁衍之义。如东汉画像石的扁鹊行医针砭图，提示了鸟图腾与医药之间的特殊关系；鸟首人身的"句芒"，为东方木神，主司生机，能增寿延年；"玄鸟贻卵"寓含生育繁殖，玄鸟即燕，后世民俗中常以燕子指代生育之喜。

## Bird totem and medicine

　　The ancient people regarded bird as totem and believed that bird could dispel diseases, promote longevity for being immortal. GE Hong's *Baopuzi* (《抱朴子》*Inner Treatise*) in the Eastern Jin Dynasty recorded "thousand-year-old birds, long-lived birds with human head and bird body, all have long life", which signified birth, health, and longevity. The special relationship between bird totem and medicine is pointed out in Bianque's stone portrait performing stone needle in the Eastern Han Dynasty. Legendary "Goumang" with bird head and human body is the Oriental Wood God, dominating vitality and life. The story "black bird spreading egg" implies reproduction and birth, and black bird particularly refers to the swallow, which represents happiness of birth in folk culture later.

# 3

# 针、砭、灸的发源地
## Birthplaces of needle, stone-needle and moxibustion

　　虽然针灸的创始者至今无定论,有关针灸空间地理上的起源却有明确文献记载。中医学最早的经典著作《黄帝内经》记载,华夏大地东、西、南、北、中央不同的地域因素,形成生活方式、饮食习惯的差异,并导致人群体质、疾病的不同,从而产生了不同的治疗方法。砭石起源于东方,九针起源于南方,药物起源于西方,艾灸起源于北方,导引按跷起源于中央。

Although the initiator of acupuncture and moxibustion therapies is inconclusive till now, their origins in space and geography have clear and definite records in some ancient documents. For instance, in book *Huangdi Neijing*, the earliest classical works on TCM, it is recorded that the territorial factor including the east, west, south, north and the center of China, and different personal life styles and diet habits generally result in a variety of physical constitutions and clinical conditions, hence producing different therapeutic methods. The Bian-stone originated from the east, the nine types of needles generated in the south, the herbal medicines derived from the west, the moxibustion stemed from the north, and the Daoist breathing exercise and massage were created from the center of ancient China.

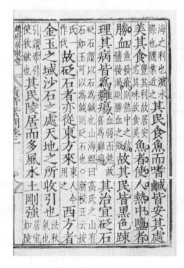
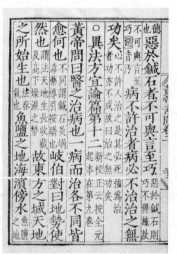

◇砭石起源地文字记载
引自《素问·异法方宜论》,明嘉靖赵康王朱厚煜居敬堂刻本,中国中医科学院图书馆藏

Written words about the area of origin of Bian-stone
Quoted from *Suwen: Yifa Fangyi Lun* (《素问·异法方宜论》*On Variation of Methods in Accordance with Geographical Locations of Suwen*), Jujingtang block-printed edition of ZHU Hou-yu (Prince of Zhao Kang)'s Mansion in the Emperor Jiajing Regime of the Ming Dynasty Preserved in the Library of CACMS

# 4

## 以石为针到针石并用

From taking stone as an acupuncture needle to joint application of metal needle and stone-needle

　　针与砭形制不同,起源地有别。一般认为,针由砭石发展而来,在金属针发明之前,古人用石器进行砭刺等外治疗法,如梁代全元起说,"砭石者,是古外治之法,……古来未能铸铁,故用石为针,故名为针石"。此外,考古发现的砭石亦可印证,如 1963 年内蒙古多伦县头道洼新石器时代遗址出土的砭石。

　　除了以砭石为针具,古人还使用竹针、陶针等。随着金属冶炼技术的出现和发展,古人制造出青铜针、铁针、金银针等。1978 年内蒙古达拉特旗发现一枚战国至西汉年间的青铜砭针,形状与内蒙古头道洼出土的砭石相似。然而,金属针具的出现并未完全取代砭石,后者在相当长的一段时间内依然被使用。

The needle and stone-needle are different in the shape, manufacturing technique and source place. Generally, it is held that the acupuncture needle is developed from Bian-stone. Before invention of metal needle, ancient Chinese used Bian-stone as a tool of the external medical therapy. In the Liang Dynasty, QUAN Yuan-qi said, "the Bian-stone is employed for external treatment of disorders. ... In the ancient times, the iron could not be manufactured, so, the sharp stone was used as an acupuncture needle. It is thus named as Bian-stone or stone-needle". Additionally, the Bian-stone discovered in an archeological study also confirms this fact. For example, in 1963, a Bian-stone was unearthed in Toudaowa of Duolun County of Inner Mongolia Autonomous Region which is the ruins of the New Stone Age.

Apart from stone-needle, ancient Chinese often used bamboo needles, clay-made needles, etc. as medical tools. Along with the appearance

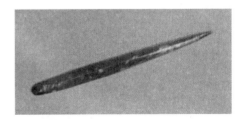

◇战国至西汉年间的青铜砭针

长 4.6cm,内蒙古达拉特旗出土

Bronze Bian-needle used from the Warring States period to the Western Han Dynasty
4.6cm in length, unearthed in the Da La Te Qi (County) of Inner Mongolia Autonomous Region

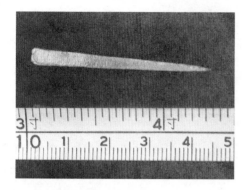

◇新石器时期的砭石

长 4.5cm，一端为四棱形可用来放血，一边为扁平
的刃可用来切开脓疡；内蒙古多伦县头道洼出土

Stone-needles of the New Stone Age
4.5cm in length, one-end being in four-edged shape, used
for bleeding, and the other end being an ancipital blade
used for cutting abscess open; unearthed in Toudaowa of
Duolun County of Inner Mongolia Autonomous Region

and development of metal smelting techniques, the ancients made bronze needles, iron needles, gold needles, silver needles, etc. In 1978, a piece of bronze-made needle from the period between the Warring-states and the Western Han Dynasty was found in Dalate Qi (County) of Inner Mongolia. This bronze needle is in a shape similar to the stone-needle unearthed from the above mentioned Toudaowa. However, stone-needle was not replaced completely by the metal needle at that time, and was still applied in a rather long period of time in ancient China.

# 5

# 火、艾与灸
## Fire, moxa and moxibustion

灸,《说文解字》言"灸者,灼也"。灸,其实就是烧灼,与火的应用有关。古人在煨火取暖时,由于偶然被火烧灼身体某处而解除了病痛,从而得到了烧灼可以防治疾病的启示。而艾草在古代常被作为辟邪、避瘟、避晦之物,可见其"纯阳之性"。将纯阳之艾燃火烧灼体表特定部位而保健、治病,从而诞生出了"艾灸"。《本草纲目》载艾叶"取太阳真火,可以回垂绝元阳。……灸之则透诸经,而治百种病邪,起沉疴之人为康泰,其功亦大矣"。

《孟子》一书有"七年之疾,而寻三年之艾"的记载。此处的"三年之艾"指陈年之艾,可见艾灸之法治疗疾病在先秦时期已较为普遍。《黄帝内经》《史记·扁鹊仓公列传》中灸法运用相当广泛,出土经脉文献《阴阳十一脉灸经》《足臂十一脉灸经》中论述每条脉的内容最后均有"皆灸某某脉",充分表明灸法已经与经脉产生了密切关联。

According to *Shuowen Jiezi* (《说文解字》*Explaining Graphs and Analyzing Characters*), the word "moxibustion" actually means "scorching", and is in relation with the application of fire. This probably comes from an enlightenment of indisposition relief by cauterization, that is, when the ancients were making a fire for keeping warmth, an ailment was unexpectedly relieved by an accident scorching of some portions of the body. In Chinese ancient times, the moxa-wood was frequently considered an object for counteracting evil spirits and avoiding acute communicable diseases, bad luck, etc., and

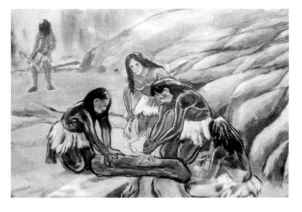

◇钻木取火
摄于湖南中医药大学针灸陈列馆

Drilling wood to make fire
Photographed in the Museum of Acupuncture and Moxibustion of Hunan University of TCM

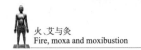

has a "nature of pure yang". When ignited to apply to a certain part of the human body, it could function well in health preservation and cure of disease, leading to the birth of moxibustion.

As those recorded in ancient Classic *Bencao Gangmu* that the Chinese mugwort leaf getting genuine fire from the sun, is able to restore yuanyang (kidney yang of TCM) from collapse... If it is ignited to apply to the body surface, the related meridians will be dredged. As a result, a lot of clinical problems would be cured, and some patients with chronic conditions would become healthy again. Thus, moxibustion therapy has an important role in clinical practice. It was recorded in book *Mengzi* (《孟子》*Mencius*) that "for treatment of a 7 years' disease, we had better to search for a moxa wood preserved for over 3 years", indicating a relatively wider application of moxibustion in clinical practice in the pre-Qin Dynasty period. Moxibustion was also frequently mentioned in books like *Huangdi Neijing* and *Shiji: Bianque Canggong Liezhuan* (《史记·扁鹊仓公列传》 *Records of Grand Historians Biographies of Bianque and Canggong*). While in the unearthed meridian documents such as *Yinyang Shiyi Mai Jiujing* and *Zubi Shiyi Mai Jiujing*, each meridian discussed is followed by that "moxibustion is applicable for certain problems". All those suggest a close correlation between moxibustion and meridians.

◇艾叶的记载

引自《本草纲目》，清顺治 14 年丁酉（1657）张朝璘刻本

中国中医科学院针灸研究所针灸博物馆藏

Record of moxa leaf

Cited from *Bencao Gangmu*, ZHANG Chao-lin's block-printed edition from the Emperor Shunzhi regime of the Qing Dynasty (1657)

Preserved by the Museum of Acupuncture and Moxibustion of the Institute of Acupuncture and Moxibustion, China Academy of Chinese Medical Sciences (CACMS)

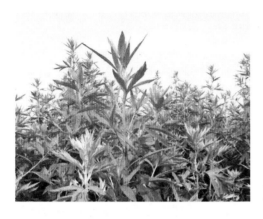

◇新鲜艾叶

摄于湖北省蕲春县

Fresh moxa leaf
Photographed in Qichun County of Hubei Province

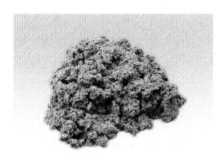

◇艾绒

Moxa wool

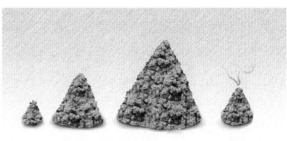

◇艾炷

Moxa cone

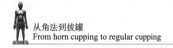

# 6

# 从角法到拔罐
From horn cupping to regular cupping

角法，是在刺破脓肿后用兽角（动物犄角）来吸拔脓疮、吸除脓血的外治法，有着悠久历史。早在《五十二病方》中就有运用角法治疗牡痔的记载，"牡痔居窍旁，大者如枣，小者如枣核者，方：以小角角之，如熟二斗米顷，而张角，系以小绳，剖以刀"。后世发展为火罐疗法，罐具亦由兽角逐步发展为竹筒、陶罐，乃至现代的玻璃罐等，治疗病种亦由痈肿脓疡演变为内外妇儿各科疾病。如晋代葛洪《肘后备急方》中所载角法，即用竹筒拔吸病痛处。

The "Jiaofa" (horn-cupping), an external remedy for sucking pus blood of a pricked fester by using a beast's horn, was once employed early in ancient China. Long ago, horn cupping was recorded in the book *Wushier Bingfang*: at the external hemorrhoids are often seen clearly around the anus, being like a jujube for the bigger one, or like a jujube pit for the smaller one. When treated, the small one is treated directly by sucking it with a small horn for a time span as about that two Dou (a measure of rice in ancient China) of rice is well cooked, followed by removing the horn forcefully; while the bigger one is treated by cupping first with a Zhang Jiao (made by the horn of ox, sheep, or deer), followed by ligature with a thin thread and cutting with a knife. Along with the unceasing development of medical practice, the "animal's horn" was gradually evolved into bamboo cup, clay cup, and the current glass cup, etc. The indications were evolved from abscess gradually to many kinds of clinical problems covering the internal medicine, surgery, gynecology, etc. GE Hong of the Jin Dynasty made a description about "Jiaofa" (horn-method) in his book *Zhouhou Beiji Fang*, "sucking the diseased site with a bamboo tube".

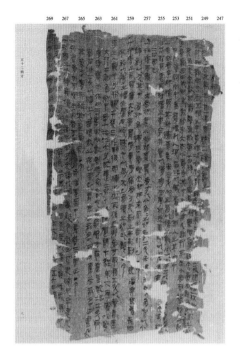

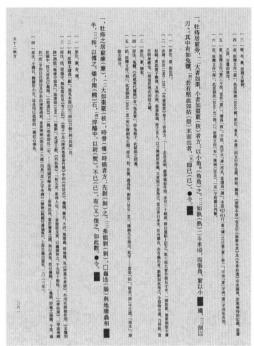

◇"角法"图版和释文注释

引自《长沙马王堆汉墓简帛集成》（裘锡圭主编,湖南省博物馆,复旦大学出土文献与古文字研究中心编纂,中华书局,2014年6月）

Picture and legend of "Jiaofa" (horn-cupping)
Quoted from book *Changsha Mawangdui Hanmu Jianbo Jicheng* (《长沙马王堆汉墓简帛集成》*Collection of Bamboo slips and Silk from Han Tomb at Mawangdui, Changsha*) (Editor-in-chief QIU Xi-gui, the Museum of Hunan Province, compiled by the Research Center of the Unearthed Literature and Ancient Characters, Fudan University, published by Zhonghua Book Company in June, 2014)

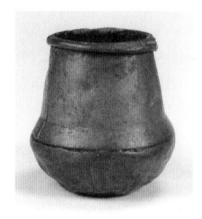

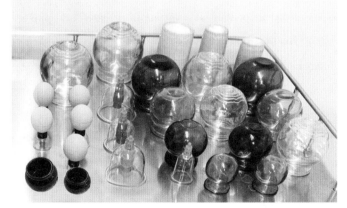

◇紫铜火罐

清代制造,陕西医史博物馆藏

Red copper cup
Made in the Qing Dynasty, collected by the
Medical History Museum of Shaanxi

◇现代常用罐具

Common modern cups

# 7

# 战国名医秦越人
QIN Yue-ren, a famous physician of the Warring States period

秦越人，又被人尊称为"扁鹊"，渤海郡鄚州（今河北任丘）人，战国时期的医学家。他学医于长桑君，精通内、外、妇产、小儿、五官、针灸等各科，特别在望诊和切脉方面有高深的造诣，医名甚著。《史记·扁鹊仓公列传》《战国策》里载其传记和病案，并推崇为脉学的倡导者。相传《黄帝八十一难经》（简称《难经》）也为秦越人所作，是中医学不可多得的理论著作之一。后因医治秦武王病，被秦国太医令李醯妒忌杀害。

QIN Yue-ren, courtesy name "Bianque", a native of Maozhou of Bohai Jun (currently, Renqiu County of Hebei Province) was a famous physician of the Warring States period. He was proficient in many disciplines inluding internal medicine, surgery, gynecology and obstetrics, pediatrics, ophthalmology and otorhinolaryngology, acupuncture-moxibustion, etc. with profound attainments especially at inspection of a variety of diseases and pulse taking. His biography and case study were included in *Shiji: Bianque Canggong Liezhuan* and *Zhanguo Ce* (《战 国 策》 *Strategies of the Warring States*), and he was highly praised as the pioneer of Chinese sphygmology. According to legend, *Huangdi Bashiyi Nanjing*, which is often referred to simply as *Nanjing*, with its authorship ascribed *to* QIN Yue-ren, is one of the exceptional medical theoretical book on TCM. Unfortunately QIN Yue-ren was killed by LI Xi (Director of Imperial Medical Bureau) who envied QIN's successfully curing King Wu's disease of the Qin Dynasty.

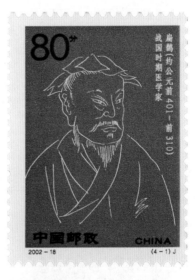

◇扁鹊邮票

中国古代科学家邮票，2002 年 8 月 20 日影雕版

A stamp for memorizing Bianque Stamps (photocopied carving edition) for memorizing ancient Chinese scientists (August 20, 2002)

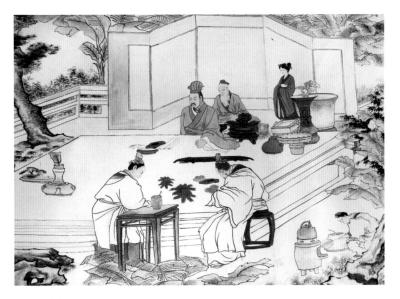

◇扁鹊诊病疗疾图

　摄于河北省内邱县神头村

A picture of Bianque treating a patient
Photographed from Shentou Village of Neiqiu County of Hebei Province

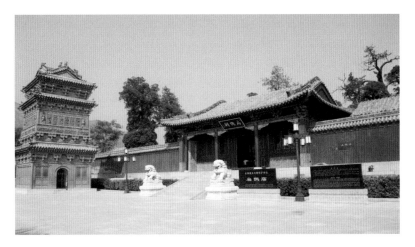

◇扁鹊祠

　摄于河北省内邱县神头村

Bianque's Memorial Temple
Taken from Shentou Village of Neiqiu County of Hebei Province

## 扁鹊治虢太子尸厥

　　有一次,扁鹊路过虢国,见那里的百姓举行祈福消灾的仪式,就上前询问,宫中喜好方术的侍从说,太子已死半日。扁鹊问明情况,认为太子患的只是一种突然昏倒不省人事的"尸厥"症,鼻息微弱,像死去一样,便亲去察看诊治。

　　诊察之后,扁鹊叫弟子子阳在石上磨针,在太子头顶中央凹陷处的百会穴扎了一针。过一会儿,太子就苏醒过来。接着叫弟子子豹在太子两胁下做药熨疗法。不久,太子就能坐起来。再服 20 天的汤以调补阴阳,虢太子就完全恢复了健康。从此以后,天下人传言扁鹊能"起死回生",但扁鹊却否认说,他并不能救活死人,只不过能把应当救活的人的病治愈罢了。

## Bianque's treatment of prince's corpse-like syncope

　　On one occasion, when Bianque passed by the Guo State, he saw people there holding a ceremony of praying for good fortune and disaster relief. He went up and inquired. The palace attendant answered that the prince had been dead for half a day. Bianque inquired about the situation, believing that the prince had suffered from only a sudden coma, "corpse-like syncope". He examined the prince and found that he still had feeble breathing and decided to treat him.

　　Bianque asked his student Ziyang to sharpen the needle on the stone first and treated the prince by puncturing a point of Baihui (GV 20) in the depression of the center of the vertex with the needle. After a while, the prince came back to his consciousness. Then Bianque asked his another student Zibao to apply a therapy of hot medicated compress along both sides of the hypochondrium of the Prince. Soon the prince could sit up. Bianque then prescribed some herbal medicine for regulation of yin-yang. After taking the herbal decoction for 20 days, the prince was cured. From then on, everyone said that Bianque could "bring the dead back to life", but Bianque denied that he could not save the dead, but could only treat the disease of the patient who should be saved.

# 8

# 最早的针灸医案
## The earliest medical case record of acupuncture and moxibustion

西汉司马迁的《史记·扁鹊仓公列传》所载仓公的诊籍是历史上最早的医案记载。仓公 25 个病案中,有 15 个进行了治疗,其中有两个使用针刺,两个使用灸法,其余均为药物疗法。从治疗部位来看,有 3 个为具体经脉,1 个为相应体表部位。这是现存最早的针灸医案。

The diagnosis records of medical cases described in SIMA Qian's book *Shiji: Bianque Canggong Liezhuan* in the Western Han Dynasty are the earliest medical report in Chinese history. Among the 25 cases of Canggong, 15 had received treatment, including two cases treated with acupuncture, two treated with moxibustion, and the rest treated with medicinal herbs. In regard of the treated areas of the body, three cases involved specific meridians, and one involved meridian-related body surface. This is the extant earliest medical case record on acupuncture and moxibustion.

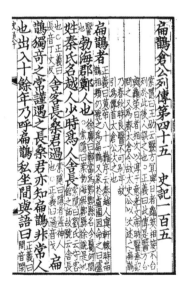

◇《史记·扁鹊仓公传》书影
**影宋本,日本刊本**

Photocopy of *Shiji Bianque Canggong Liezhuan*
A photograph of Song Dynasty's copy, Japanese block-printed version

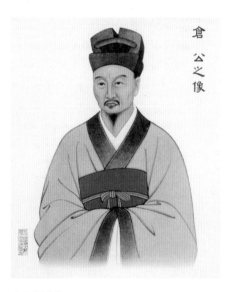

◇仓公画像
**宋大仁绘**

Canggong's portrait
Painted by SONG Da-ren

## 仓公与缇萦救父

　　仓公,姓淳于,名意,临淄人,因曾任齐国太仓长,故史称太仓公,简称仓公,是西汉初期著名医家。仓公有 5 个女儿,缇萦排行第五,自幼聪慧、孝亲。淳于意因得罪权贵,"以刑罪当传至长安",坐肉刑(诸如脸上刺字、割去鼻子、砍去左足或右足等),姐妹 5 人围在父亲身边流泪,却无力替父鸣冤。淳于意悲愤地仰天长叹:"生子不生男,缓急非有益。"小女缇萦听此言悲伤痛心,自问:"为什么女儿就不能像男儿一样为父伸冤辩诬?"她痛下决心要救父免罪脱刑,遂伴父来到长安,冒死入宫上书云:"女愿意被收为官府的奴婢,替父赎罪,使父亲能改过自新。"缇萦舍身救父的孝义行为,深深打动了汉文帝,他顿生怜悯之情,遂下诏免了淳于意的肉刑。后来汉文帝诏令废除肉刑,揭开了中国法律史上重要的一页,缇萦也谱写了一曲千古传唱的孝义之歌。

## Canggong and Ti Ying saving her father

　　Canggong, surname CHUNYU, given name Yi, born in Linzi, once was appointed as a Taicang official of the former Qi state, so he was called Taicang Gong, Cang Gong for short. He was a famous doctor in the early Western Han Dynasty and had five daughters, of whom Tiying was the youngest. She was intelligent and filial. When CHUNYU Yi accidentally offended the influential officials, "the crime of punishment should be passed to Chang'an". He would be sentenced to corporal punishment (such as stabbing his face, cutting off his nose, cutting off his left foot or right foot, etc.). The five sisters surrounded their father and wept, but could not complain for his father. CHUNYU Yi sighed with grief and indignation: "It's a pity I have no son. Who can help me when I am now in danger?" Tiying, the little girl felt so sad on hearing this. She asked herself, "Why can't daughters justify their father like boys?" After determining to save her father from punishment, she accompanied him to Chang'an and ventured to write in the palace: "I am a girl willing to be a servant of the government to make atonement for my father, so that my father can mend his ways". Tiying's filial piety to save her father deeply touched Emperor Wendi of the Han Dynasty. He felt pity for him, and then ordered the abolition of corporal punishment, which opened an important page in the history of Chinese law. Tiying also wrote a song of filial piety and righteousness that has been praised for thousands of years.

# 9

# 出土西汉经脉文献

Meridian literature of Western Han Dynasty unearthed

关于经脉理论的起源问题一直处于历史的迷雾与纷争之中。20世纪70年代以前，《黄帝内经》所载的经络理论是我们能够见到的最早资料。1973年长沙马王堆三号汉墓出土了一批医学相关文献，其中有些与经脉理论密切相关，命名为《足臂十一脉灸经》《阴阳十一脉灸经》（有甲本、乙本之分，内容有个别文字出入），后者在1983年湖北江陵张家山出土竹简《脉书》中亦有基本相同内容（即《阴阳十一脉灸经》丙本）。这些出土经脉文献展现了经脉理论的早期面貌，为深入了解经络理论的形成与发展提供了非常宝贵的资料。

The origin of the theory of meridians has always been in the mists and disputation. Before 1970s, the descriptions about meridian-collateral theory recorded in *Huangdi Neijing* were the earliest materials seen up to now. Among the medical literature unearthed from Changsha Mawangdui Tomb of the Han Dynasty in 1973, the meridian-collateral theory related data were *Zubi Shiyi Mai Jiujing* (《足臂十一脉灸经》*Moxibustion Classic on Eleven Meridians of Legs and Arms*) and *Yinyang Shiyi Mai Jiujing* (《阴阳十一脉灸经》*Moxibustion Classic on Eleven Meridians of Yin-yang*), the latter contains Copy A and Copy B, being different only in a few words. The latter also contains some contents similar to those in *Maishu* (《脉书》*A Book on Pulse Condition*, i.e., *Copy C of book A Book of Yinyang Shiyi Mai Jiujing*) written on bamboo-slips unearthed from Zhangjiashan Tomb in Jiangling County of Hubei Province in 1983. These unearthed literatures show the early feature of meridian theory and provide a very valuable historical information for understanding the formation and development of the meridian-collateral theory.

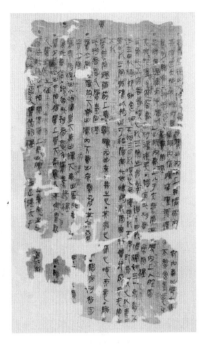
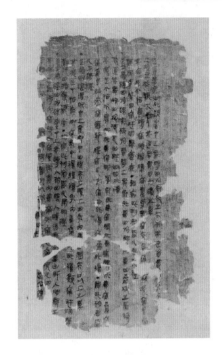

◇马王堆帛书《足臂十一脉灸经》
湖南省博物馆藏

Mawangdui Tomb's silk-book *Zubi Shiyi Mai Jiujing*
Collected by the Museum of Hunan Province

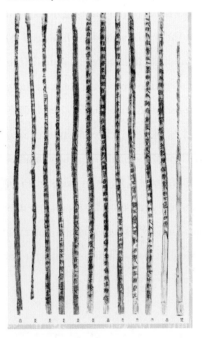
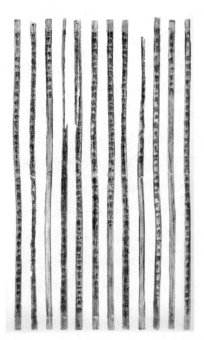

◇张家山汉简《脉书》
湖北省荆州市博物馆藏

The Han Dynasty's bamboo-slips *Maishu* uncovered in *Zhangjiashan*
Collected by Jingzhou Museum of Hubei Province

**马王堆出土医学文献**

　　1973 年，长沙马王堆三号汉墓中出土了大量医学相关文献，基本涵盖了《汉书·艺文志》对"方技"的分类，即属于医经类的《足臂十一脉灸经》《阴阳十一脉灸经》《脉法》《阴阳脉死候》，属于经方类的《五十二病方》，属于房中类的《杂疗方》《养生方》《十问》《天下至道谈》《合阴阳》，属于神仙类的《去谷食气》《胎产书》《杂禁方》《导引图》。这些文献均不见于历代书目著录，亦未见任何古籍称引。可见，当时民间业已存在较多的同类文献，医学相关知识在民间流传亦较为普遍。凭借这些出土医学文献，可以构建较以往更为丰满而鲜活的早期医学图景。

## Medical literature unearthed in Mawangdui

　　In 1973, a large number of medical documents were unearthed from Changsha Mawangdui tomb of the Han Dynasty, which basically covered the classification of "Prescription Skills" in *Hanshu: Yiwen Zhi* (《汉书·艺文志》*History of the Han Dynasty: Records of Library Classification*). The meridian-collateral theory related data were *Zubi Shiyi Mai Jiujing*, *Yinyang Shiyi Mai Jiujing*, *Maifa* (《脉法》*Methods of Pulse Diagnosis*), and *Yinyang Mai Sihou* (《阴阳脉死候》*Yin-yang Pulse for Death Diagnosis*), Classic formula related was *Wushier Bingfang*, sexual health care related included *Za Liao Fang* (《杂疗方》*Prescriptions for Different Treatment*), *Yangsheng Fang* (《养生方》*Prescriptions for Health Preservation*), *Shi Wen* (《十问》*Ten Questions*), *Tianxia Zhidao Tan* (《天下至道谈》*Lectures on the Super Tao in the World*), *He Yin Yang* (《合阴阳》*Methods of Intercourse between Yin and Yang*) celestial classified ones were *Qugu Shiqi* (《去谷食气》*Qigong Exercise and Fasting for Health Preservation*), *Taichan Shu* (《胎产书》*Book of Pregnancy and Obstetric*), *Zajin Fang* (《杂禁方》*Methods of Sexual Activities*) and *Daoyin Tu* (《导引图》*Picture of Physical and Breathing Exercises*).

　　These literature data had neither been recorded in bibliographies of the past dynasties, nor cited in any classics, which indicated that at that time many similar books existed, and medical related knowledge was quite popular. With these unearthed medical literature, we are able to draw a more colorful and vivid medical picture of the early stage currently than before.

# 10

# 《五十二病方》中的砭灸内容
Contents of stone-needle and moxibustion in book *Wushier Bingfang* (*Prescriptions for Fifty-two Diseases*)

马王堆出土医学文献《五十二病方》不属于经脉文献,而是论述各种疾病的具体治疗方法,主要为药物疗法,其中也有较少病例使用砭石与灸法,并无针法。如书中记载运用砭刺治疗癫病,运用灸法治疗疣、痔、癫、牡痔、白处等病。出土经脉文献《足臂十一脉灸经》《阴阳十一脉灸经》中亦只提及灸法。《五十二病方》中砭石与灸法使用的部位多描述为相应体表部位或病变部位,只有一处提及"太阴、太阳",并未出现具体腧穴名称。

*Wushier Bingfang* uncovered from Mawangdui tomb does not belong to the meridian literature, and rather, is a book expounding concrete pharmacotherapies for a variety of clinical conditions, mainly involving medications, but also containing fewer cases treated with stone-needle (without any needling methods) and moxibustion. In the book, the stone needle was applied to treat edema of scrotum, and moxibustion applied to treat problems like wart, dripping of urine, edema of scrotum, hemorrhoids, etc. In the unearthed book *Zubi Shiyi Mai Jiujing* and *Yinyang Shiyi Mai Jiujing*, only moxibustion is mentioned. In *Wushier Bingfang*, the stimulated sites of the body for stone-needle and moxibustion described are some superficial portions or the affected spots of the body without concrete acupoint names, and there is only one sentence referring "Taiyin" and "Taiyang".

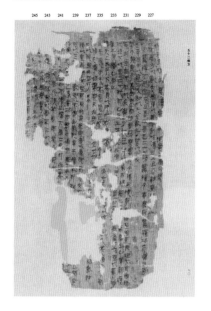

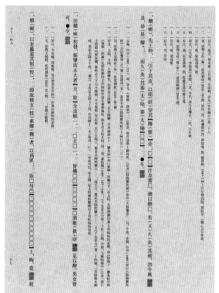

◇"砭法"图版和释文注释

引自《长沙马王堆汉墓简帛集成》(裘锡圭主编,湖南省博物馆,复旦大学出土文献与古文字研究中心编纂,中华书局,2014年6月)

Picture and interpretation and commentary of "Bian Fa" (Bian-stone needling)

Quoted from *Changsha Mawangdui Hanmu Jianbo Jicheng* (Editor-in-chief QIU Xi-gui, Museum of Hunan Province, compiled by the Research Center for the Unearthed Literature and Ancient Characters of Fudan University, published by Zhonghua Book Company in June 2014)

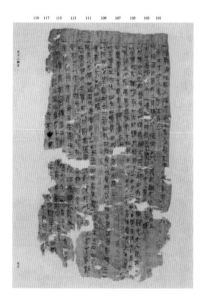

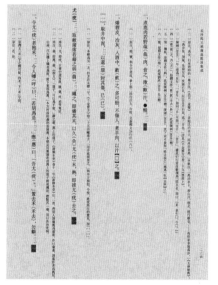

◇"灸法"图版和释文注释

引自《长沙马王堆汉墓简帛集成》(裘锡圭主编,湖南省博物馆,复旦大学出土文献与古文字研究中心编纂,中华书局,2014年6月)

Picture and interpretation and commentary of "Jiu Fa" (Moxibustion)

Quoted from *Changsha Mawangdui Hanmu Jianbo Jicheng* (Editor-in-chief QIU Xi-gui, Museum of Hunan Province, compiled by the Research Center for the Unearthed Literature and Ancient Characters of Fudan University, published by Zhonghua Book Company in June 2014)

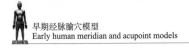
# 11

## 早期经脉腧穴模型
### Early human meridian and acupoint models

1993 年,四川绵阳双包山二号西汉墓出土了一木人模型,高 28.1cm,木胎,体表髹黑漆,裸体直立,手臂伸直,掌心向前,体表绘有纵形红线 19 条,并未标注穴位,发掘者命名为"人体经脉漆雕"。

2012—2013 年间,四川成都金牛区天回镇(当地俗称"老官山")西汉墓出土一木制"人体经穴漆木俑"。该人像高 14cm,标记红色粗线 22 条,阴刻白色细线 29 条,黄白色腧穴点 119 个,及"心""肺""肾""盆"等阴刻小字。其年代略晚于双包山经脉漆雕,是迄今为止我国发现的最早、最完整的经穴人体模型。

In 1993, a wooden manikin was unearthed from the No.2 Western Han tomb in Shuangbaoshan, Mianyang City of Sichuan Province in China. This manikin is 28.1cm in height, coated with black lacquer, with the palm center facing forward and with 19 longitudinal red strips painted on the nude body surface, but without acupoint labelling. The excavators called it "black-lacquered figure with meridians" (meridian-manikin).

From 2012 to 2013, a "lacquered wooden figure with acupoints" (acupoint-manikin) was unearthed from the tomb of the Western Han Dynasty in Tianhui Township (nicknamed "*Laoguan Mountain*" by local people) of Jinniu District, Chengdu City, Sichuan Province. This acupoint-manikin is 14cm in height, marked with 22 red thick strips, 29 intagliated white thin strips, 119 yellowish white acupoints, as well as intagliated small characters as "heart", "lung", "kidney" and "pelvic". It is a little later than "Shuangbaoshan meridian-manikin" and is the earliest and most complete human acupoint model in China.

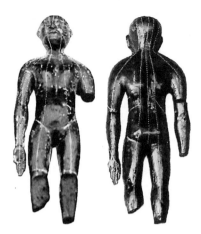

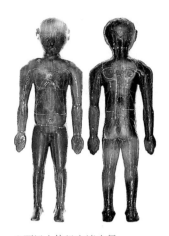

◇西汉人体经脉漆雕

四川绵阳双包山汉墓出土，四川省绵阳市博物馆藏

Western Han lacquered meridian manikin
Unearthed from the Western Han tomb in Shuangbaoshan of Mianyang City, Sichuan Province, and collected by the Museum of Mianyang City, Sichuan Province

◇西汉人体经穴漆木俑

四川天回镇汉墓出土，四川省成都博物馆藏

Western Han lacquered wooden acupoint manikin
Unearthed from the Han tomb in Tianhui Township of Sichuan Province, and collected by the Museum of Chengdu City, Sichuan Province

 ## 古代巫蛊术之中的桐人、木偶

　　绵阳双包山汉墓出土的人体漆雕，在古代被称作桐人、木偶，与巫术、医学密切相关。《汉书·江充传》记载了江充利用汉武帝畏恶巫蛊的心理，在太子宫中埋桐木人，以嫁祸卫皇后和戾太子刘据。《三辅旧事》记载："江充为桐人，长尺，以针刺其腹，埋太子宫中。充晓医术，因言其事。"江充通晓医术，针刺桐人的腹部要害之处以致人死地，从而嫁祸他人。此外，还有徐秋夫针灸疗鬼的故事也是与桐人、木偶相关。《南史·张邵传》记载，一鬼患腰痛难忍，求治于徐秋夫，鬼变为刍人（即桐人、木偶之类），徐秋夫在刍人上施行针灸治疗而病愈。

## Wooden (paulownia) manikin, puppet in ancient witchcraft

　　The lacquered wooden manikin unearthed from the Han tomb in Shuangbaoshan, Mianyang was closely related to witchcraft and medicine. *Hanshu: Jiangchong Zhuan* (《汉书·江充传》 *History of the Han Dynasty: Biography of JIANG Chong*) records that JIANG Chong buried a wooden manikin in the palace to shift the misfortune onto the empress and prince because he knew that the Emperor Wudi of the Han Dynasty psychologically was afraid of witchcraft. *Sanfu Jiushi* (《三辅旧事》 *Old Stories of the Three Regions*) recorded "JIANG Chong was good at medicine and able to puncture the vital points of the abdomen of the wooden manikin to cause death and bring misfortune onto the others". In addition, XU Qiu-fu's story of treating ghosts with acupuncture was also related to puppet, wooden manikin. *Nanshi: Zhangshao Zhuan* (《南史·张邵传》 *History of the Southern Dynasty: Biography of Zhang Shao*) said that a ghost was suffering from lower back pain, asking XU Qiu-fu for treatment. After the change from a ghost into a manikin (wooden manikin, puppet), XU Qiu-fu treated and cured the manikin with acupuncture.

# 12

# 《黄帝内经》与针灸学理论体系

## *Huangdi Neijing* (*The Yellow Emperor's Inner Classic*) and the theoretical system of acupuncture and moxibustion

　　《黄帝内经》(简称《内经》),是我国现存最早的医学理论著作。《内经》原书 18 卷,其中《素问》和《灵枢》各 9 卷,是战国至秦汉医家将历代医学经验收集、整理而成的。《内经》中关于疾病的治疗,使用药方仅 13 首,绝大部分采用针灸治疗。《内经》近一半的篇幅论述针灸学的有关内容,特别是《灵枢》大部分篇幅阐述针灸内容,主要包括经络理论、腧穴理论、刺灸理论、针灸治疗等,基本构建了针灸学理论体系。

*Huangdi Neijing or Neijing* (《黄帝内经》*The Yellow Emperor's Inner Classic*) is the first and the earliest extant works on Chinese medical theory in China. The original book is composed of 18 volumes, including 9 volumes of *Suwen* (《素问》*Basic Questions*) and 9 volumes of *Lingshu* (《灵枢》*Miraculous Pivot*). It was completed by ancient Chinese medical specialists from the Warring States period to the Qin and Han Dynasties on the basis of systematical collection and sorting of the medical literature in the past successive dynasties. In regard to the treatment of diseases in book *Huangdi Neijing*, only 13 formulae of herbal medicines are recorded and majority of the diseases are treated by using acupuncture and moxibustion. Nearly half of the contents of *Huangdi Neijing* involves acupuncture and moxibustion, particularly in *Lingshu* which mainly focuses on the theory of meridian-collaterals, theory of acupoints, theory of acupuncture needling and moxibustion skills, acupuncture-moxibustion therapy, constituting the basic theoretical system of acupuncture and moxibustion medicine.

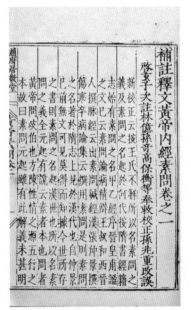

◇《素问》书影
明赵府居敬堂刻本,中国中医科学院图书馆藏

Photocopy of *Suwen*
Zhao-mansion's Jujingtang block-printed edition of *Suwen* in the Ming Dynasty, collected by the Library of CACMS

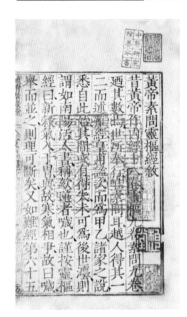

 ◇《灵枢》书影

明赵府居敬堂刻本,中国中医科学院针灸研究所针灸博物馆藏

Photocopy of *Lingshu*

Zhao-mansion's Jujingtang block-printed edition of *Lingshu* in the Ming Dynasty, collected by the Chinese Museum of Acupuncture and Moxibustion, Institute of Acupuncture and Moxibustion, CACMS

## 《黄帝内经》与黄帝有关吗?

　　《黄帝内经》是否为黄帝所著,或出于黄帝时代?后世多数医家认为,《黄帝内经》并非出于黄帝岐伯之手,也不是黄帝时代的著作,而是托名于黄帝,《黄帝内经》之前冠以"黄帝"二字,仅仅是为了"溯源崇本"。因黄帝是华夏民族崇拜的祖先,故先秦时期的一切文物制度、发明创造、书籍名称,多冠以黄帝。这反映了当时的崇古思想已形成社会风气,溯本思源,以示学有根本。正如《淮南子》说:"世俗之人,多尊古而贱今,故为道者必托之于神农、黄帝而后能入说。"因此,《黄帝内经》冠以黄帝,其意义也是如此。

## *Is Huangdi Neijing related to Huangdi?*

　　Is *Huangdi Neijing* written by Huangdi or in the age of Huangdi? Most physicians believed that *Huangdi Neijing* was not written by Emperor and Qibo, nor was it written in the Yellow Emperor's time, but was named after Emperor Huangdi. Before *Huangdi Neijing*, it was crowned with the word "Huangdi" just to "trace back to the source and worship the original". Because Huangdi, the Yellow Emperor was the ancestor of the Chinese nation, all the cultural relics system, inventions and books in the pre-Qin period were often crowned with the title Huangdi, Yellow Emperor. This reflects the respect of ancient culture and the original source. As what is described in *Huainanzi* (《淮南子》*A Book of Philosophy* Dynasty), "People usually respect the old more than the new, the theory and study are often based on ancestors, Shennong and Huangdi". Therefore, Huangdi has been added to the name of *Huangdi Neijing*.

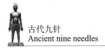

# 13

## 古代九针
### Ancient nine needles

　　九针，为九种不同形制的针具，是古代医家在长期的医疗实践活动中发展而来，首载于《灵枢·九针十二原》，篇中对九针的形制与功用有详细描述，计有镵针、员针、鍉针、员利针、铍针、锋针、大针、毫针和长针九种。但传世本未见相应的针具图，在古医籍中，最早是元代杜思敬《针经摘英集》绘有"九针图"，之后明清医家先后绘制有"九针图"。

　　The nine types of needle were developed by ancient medical experts during long-term medical practice in China. They were recorded first and described in detail in book *Lingshu: Jiuzhen Shier Yuan* (《灵枢·九针十二原》*Lingshu: Nine Needles and Twelve Primary Points*), including Chanzhen (shear needle), Yuanzhen (round-point needle), Chizhen (spoon needle), Yuanli zhen (round-sharp needle), Pizhen (stiletto needle), Fengzhen (lance needle), Dazhen (big needle), Haozhen (filiform needle) and Changzhen (long needle). But not any related pictures have been found in various versions of *Lingshu* handed down from the ancient times. In the ancient medical works, the earliest pictures of the nine classical needles were seen in *Zhenjing Zhaiying Ji* (《针经摘英集》*A Collection of Gems from Acupuncture Classic*) written by DU Si-jing of the Yuan Dynasty. Thereafter, the nine needles were drawn up successively in the Ming and Qing Dynasties.

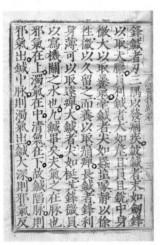 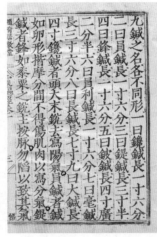

◇《灵枢》中的九针记载

明赵府居敬堂刻本，中国中医科学院图书馆藏

Recordings of nine needles in *Lingshu*
Zhao-mansion's Jujingtang block-printed edition of *Lingshu* in the Ming Dynasty, collected by the Library of CACMS

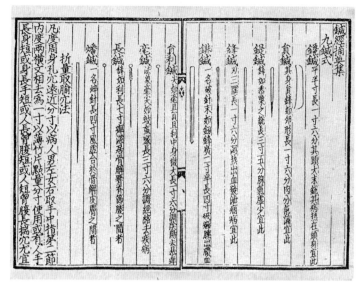

◇《针经摘英集》九针图

影印本，中国中医科学院图书馆藏

Picture of nine needles in *Zhenjing Zhaiying Ji*

Photocopy of *Zhenjing Zhaiying Ji* of the Yuan Dynasty, collected by the Library of CACMS

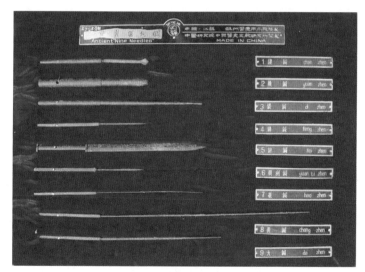

◇仿古九针模型

苏州医疗用品厂有限公司制造，中国中医科学院医史文献所监制，中国中医科学院针灸研究所针灸博物馆藏

The replicated nine needles model Manufactured by Suzhou Medical Instrument Factory Limited, supervised by the Institute for Medical History and Literature, collected by Chinese Museum of Acupuncture and Moxibustion, Institute of Acupuncture and Moxibustion, CACMS

# 14

## 汉墓金银医针
### Gold and silver acupuncture needles unearthed from Mancheng Tomb of the Han Dynasty

1968 年,在河北满城西汉中山靖王刘胜墓出土金医针 4 枚,银医针 6 枚。其中,金医针制作精细,保存完好,针体长 6.5~6.9cm,上端为方柱形的柄,比针身略粗,柄上有一小孔,计有锃针、锋针各 1 枚,毫针 2 枚;6 枚银医针都残缺,无法辨认,有 1 根可能是员针。据研究,这批金银医针与《灵枢》中《九针十二原》所述形制相似,属于两千年前遗留下来的"古九针",可认为是现存最早的针具实物。

In 1968, 4 pieces of gold acupuncture needles and 6 pieces of silver acupuncture needles were unearthed from LIU Sheng's Tomb in Mancheng County of Hebei Province (LIU Sheng: Prince Zhongshan of the Western Han Dynasty). The gold medical needles, including 1 spoon needle, 1 lance needle and 2 filiform needles, are intact and delicate in manufacture, 6.5–6.9cm in length. Its top part is a cubic handle, being slightly thicker than the needle body, and with a small hole in it. All the 6 silver medical needles are incomplete and nearly unable to be recognized. One of them is probably a round-point needle. It was thought in a study that these needles are similar in shape to those described in book *Lingshu: Jiuzhen Shier Yuan*, and should belong to the "ancient nine types of acupuncture needles" handed down to us 2,000 years ago. These medical needles could be considered to be the extant earliest acupuncture needle entities in China.

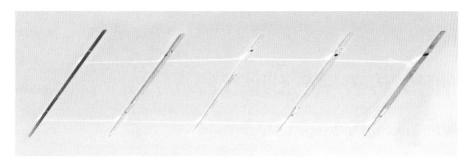

◇满城汉墓金银医针
　摄于河北省博物馆

Medical gold and silver acupuncture needles unearthed from Mancheng (County) Tomb of the Han Dynasty
Taken from the Museum of Hebei Province

 ## 中山靖王刘胜墓

　　刘胜,西汉中山靖王,系汉武帝之兄,蜀汉皇帝刘备第十三世先祖,为第一代中山国国王,死后葬于今河北满城县陵山。1968 年,解放军某部在陵山上施工,在炸掉的石头下面发现一个洞,满城汉墓由此被发现并挖掘。满城汉墓凿山为陵,为规模宏大的崖洞墓,包括西汉中山靖王刘胜墓(一号墓)及其妻窦绾墓(二号墓),葬于公元前 113—前 103 年间。墓室内部布局完全模仿墓主生前所居宫室而建,宛如一座豪华的宫殿。墓内出土大量珍贵文物,尤以墓主人的两套完整的"金缕玉衣""长信宫灯""错金博山炉"闻名海内外。上文所述之金银医针即出土于刘胜墓,引起中医针灸学界的极大关注。

## Liu Sheng's Tomb

　　LIU Sheng, emperor of Zhongshan in the Western Han Dynasty, was the brother of Wudi of the Han Dynasty, the 13th ancestor of LIU Bei (Emperor of Shu-han during the Three Kingdoms period). He was the first king of Zhongshan. After his death, he was buried in Lingshan Mountain, Mancheng County, Hebei Province. In 1968, when a PLA unit was working on the Lingshan Mountain, a hole was found beneath the blasted stone, from which the Mancheng Han Tomb was discovered and excavated. The Han tomb in Mancheng was a large-scale cliff cave tomb, including the tomb of Liu Sheng (No.1) and his wife Dou Wan (No.2), buried between 113 B.C. –103 B.C. The interior layout of the tomb was completely modeled on the palace where the tomb owner lived. It was like a luxurious palace. A large number of precious cultural relics unearthed in the tomb, especially the two complete sets of "Gold-woven jade clothes", "Palace lantern" and "Boshan incense burner inlaid with gold decorations", have been famous at home and abroad. The gold and silver needles mentioned above were unearthed in LIU Sheng's tomb, causing great concern in the field of acupuncture and moxibustion.

最早的腧穴专著《黄帝明堂经》
The earliest monograph on acupoints: *Huangdi Mingtang Jing* (*The Yellow Emperor's Classic of Acupoints*)

# 15

# 最早的腧穴专著《黄帝明堂经》
## The earliest monograph on acupoints: *Huangdi Mingtang Jing* (*The Yellow Emperor's Classic of Acupoints*)

　　《黄帝明堂经》是我国第一部针灸腧穴专书,约成书于东汉初,它汇集汉代及汉以前的大量针灸文献,主要内容包括腧穴的名称、部位、主治病症及刺灸法诸方面,惜已佚。晋代皇甫谧所著我国现存最早的针灸专著《针灸甲乙经》,即是将《素问》《针经》(即《灵枢》)、《黄帝明堂经》分类合编而成。今在俄罗斯艾尔米塔什(Ermitage)博物馆藏有三片中国和田出土的古代腧穴文献古卷子残页,据考证即为《黄帝明堂经》另一古传本残页。

*Huangdi Mingtang Jing* (《黄帝明堂经》*The Yellow Emperor's Classic of Acupoints*) is the first classical book on acupoints in China, and was completed in the primary stage of the Eastern Han Dynasty. It collected a large quantity of documents on acupuncture and moxibustion during and before the Han Dynasty. Its main contents covered the name, location and clinical indications of acupoints, and methods of needling and moxibustion. But unfortunately, this book was lost. *Zhenjiu Jiayi Jing*, the extant earliest monograph on acupuncture and moxibustion written by HUANGFU Mi in the Jin Dynasty, is composed of *Suwen* and *Zhenjing* (《针经》*Classic of Acupuncture*, i.e., *Lingshu*) and *Huangdi Mingtang Jing*. Now, in Ermitage Museum of Russia, there are 3 incomplete pages of a literature about the ancient acupoints unearthed from Hetian of Xinjiang Autonomic Region of China. It has been identified that those 3 incomplete pages are part of *Huangdi Mingtang Jing*, one of the ancient inherited books.

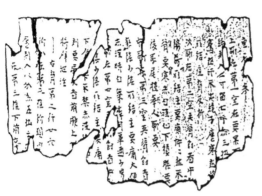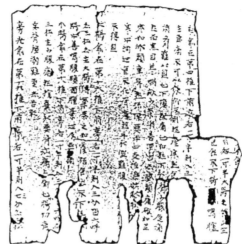

◇《黄帝明堂经》残页
俄罗斯艾尔米塔什博物馆藏

Fragments of *Huangdi Mingtang Jing*
Collected by the Ermitage Museum of Russia

 ## 书名"明堂"的由来

　　追溯古代历史，最早"明堂"二字曾是指黄帝时代的一种建筑，是黄帝测天象、观四方和举行重大政治文化活动的场所。后来，将腧穴书普遍冠以"明堂"二字，其原因可能是腧穴分属十二经与"明堂"建筑有十二宫类似。同时，每经各有五腧穴，皆自下而上依次流注，与帝王每月居一室，依次轮流居住的特点亦相类似。并且，在针灸治疗上取五腧穴的原则也与时令有关，这也符合"明堂"的特点。

## The origin of "Mingtang"

　　Tracing back to ancient history, the earliest word "Mingtang" used to refer to a building in the Yellow Emperor's time. It was the place where the Yellow Emperor surveyed the heaven, observed the Quartet and held important political and cultural activities. Later, acupoints were generally labeled as "Mingtang". The reason may be that acupoints belong to the twelve meridians, and there are twelve palaces in the building of "Mingtang"; they are similar. At the same time, there are five-Shu points in each meridian, flowing from the bottom to the top, which is similar to the Emperor's monthly in-turn residence in the palace. Moreover, the principle of selecting five-Shu points in acupuncture and moxibustion treatment is also related to the seasons, which is in accordance with the characteristics of "Mingtang".

# 16

## 《难经》与针灸
*Nanjing (Classic on Difficult Problems)* and
acupuncture-moxibustion

《黄帝八十一难经》,简称《难经》,全书以问答的形式注释了《素问》《灵枢》中的疑难,并在此基础上又有所发挥,共讨论了 81 个问题,分脉诊、经络、脏腑、腧穴、针刺及疾病等方面。书中大量关于针刺的论述是对《内经》针灸理论的补充与发展,对后世针灸医学产生了深远影响。

*Huangdi Bashiyi Nanjing* (《黄帝八十一难经》*The Yellow Emperor's Classic on 81 Difficult Medical Problems*), simplied as *Nanjing* (《难经》*Classic on Difficult Problems*), answered the medical problems listed in *Suwen* and *Lingshu*, some of which are elaborated in the contents. A total of 81 medical issues including pulse diagnosis, meridian-collaterals, Zangfu-organs, acupoints, acupuncture and various clinical conditions (or diseases) are discussed. Its expositions on acupuncture are in fact the supplement and development of the related theories in *Huangdi Neijing*, bringing about far-reaching influence on the acupuncture-moxibustin medicine of the later generations.

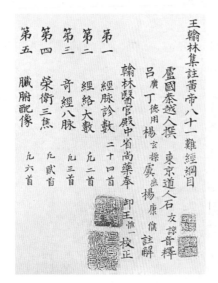

◇《集注八十一难经》书影
　古抄本,中国台北故宫博物院藏

Photograph of *Jizhu Bashiyi Nanjing* (《集注八十一难经》*Variorum on the Classics of 81 Difficult Medical Problems*)
An ancient hand-copied book, collected by the National Palace Museum of Taipei, China

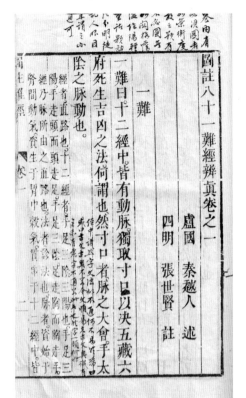

◇《图注八十一难经辨真》书影

清乾隆武林万卷堂刻本

中国中医科学院针灸研究所针灸博物馆藏

Photograph of *Tuzhu Bashiyi Nanjing Bianzhen* (《图注八十一难经辨真》*Identification on the Classics of 81 Difficult Medical Problems*) Block-printed edition from Wulin Wanjuantang, Qianlong regime of the Qing Dynasty collected by Chinese Museum of Acupuncture and Moxibustion, Institute of Acupuncture and Moxibustion, CACMS

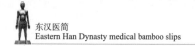

# 17

## 东汉医简

Eastern Han Dynasty medical bamboo slips

1972 年，甘肃省武威旱滩坡东汉墓出土了一批医药简牍，其中有 9 枚医简涉及针灸。医简论述了针灸治疗疾病与针灸禁忌等内容，提出根据病情取用不同腧穴组成针灸处方，按施术先后刺入不同深度，并采用不同的留针时间等。所记载的内容多未见于其他针灸著述，且腧穴名称、定位异于后世专著。此外，医简还详细记录了人生从 1~100 岁的各个年龄阶段针灸治疗时应禁忌的脏腑、部位和预后，以及针灸饮药禁忌的时日。

In 1972, some medical bamboo slips were unearthed from the Eastern Han Dynasty tomb at Hantanpo, Wuwei County of Gansu Province. Among them, 9 bamboo slips involve acupuncture and moxibustion, describing some contents about the treatment of disorders, contraindications, acupuncture prescriptions of acupoints selected according to the state of disease, different needle-insertion depths and different needle-retention time determined in the light of the needling sequence. Majority of the contents have not been found in other works on acupuncture and moxibustion up to now. Both the name and location of the applied acupoints are different from those in some monographs on acupuncture-moxibustion in the late ages. Moreover, these medical bamboo slips also expound the interrelation between the acupuncture contraindications and the patients' age-stages, and pointed out in detail the contraindications about the location of the body, organs, prognosis, and the time for patients to receive acupuncture and herbal medicine treatments from one year to 100 years in age.

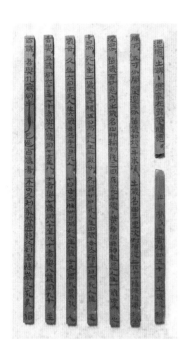

◇东汉武威医简复制品

　　中国中医科学院针灸研究所针灸博物馆藏

Replicated medical bamboo slips from Wuwei Tomb of the Eastern Han Dynasty Collected by Chinese Museum of Acupuncture and Moxibustion Institute of Acupuncture and Moxibustion, CACMS

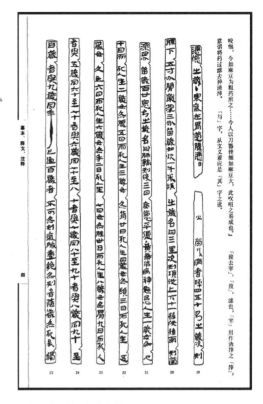

◇《武威汉代医简》书影

　　甘肃省博物馆、武威县文化馆合编，文物出版社，1975 年

Photograph of *Wuwei Handai Yijian* (《武威汉代医简》 *Medical Bamboo Slips from Wuwei Tomb of the Han Dynasty*) Collected by Museum of Gansu Province, edited jointly by Wuwei Culture Center, published by Cultural Relics Press in 1975

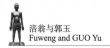

# 18

# 涪翁与郭玉
## Fuweng and GUO Yu

　　涪翁，东汉初年针灸学家。据《后汉书·郭玉传》记载，涪翁是古代一位隐姓埋名的民间医生，喜欢游历各地行医，因常在涪水边捕鱼、钓鱼而以涪翁称之。涪翁医术高明，精于针灸，遇有疾痛患者，便随时针刺施灸，几乎手到病除，撰有《针经》《诊脉法》等书，均佚。涪翁所撰的《针经》，是祖国医学第一本针灸专书。在这之前，虽《内经》有针灸论述，扁鹊等人在治病中亦运用针灸，但尚无针灸专著问世。

　　郭玉，字通直，涪翁的再传弟子，四川新都县人，生长在东汉时期，官至太医丞校尉。郭玉的医术高明，医德高尚，尤精于诊脉和针灸，切脉诊证，言之甚验，疗效也很好。

　　Fuweng was an acupuncturist in the early period of the Eastern Han Dynasty. According to the book *Hou Hanshu: Guoyu Zhuan* (《后汉书·郭玉传》*History of the Late Han Dynasty: GUO Yu's Biography*), FU Weng was a civil physician living incognito in ancient China. He liked traveling and practicing medicine everywhere. He was named as Fuweng (weng means old man in Chinese) because he frequently caught fish or went fishing in Fushui River. Fuweng was highly qualified in medical skills and proficient in acupuncture and moxibustion therapies. When meeting patients suffering from pain, he immediately employed acupuncture or moxibustion therapy to relieve it very effectively. He once wrote book *Zhenjing* (《针经》*Classic of Acupuncture*), *Zhen Mai Fa* (《诊脉法》*Methods for Pulse Taking*), etc., but all of them have been lost. His *Zhenjing* was the first monograph on acupuncture in Chinese medicine. Before then, despite of having had descriptions on acupuncture and moxibustion in *Huangdi Neijing*, and having had clinical application of these therapies to the treatment of various disorders by Bianque, et al, no monographs had been published.

　　GUO Yu, courtesy name Tongzhi, was Fuweng's second-generation disciple. He was born in Xindu County of Sichuan Province, and grew up in the Eastern Han Dynasty period. He was promoted to be "Taiyi Cheng Xiaowei" (an official) of the imperial physician academy. He was consummate in medical skills particularly in pulse-taking and acupuncture-moxibustion skills, and was noble in medical morality. He mastered pulse-taking technique and syndrome diagnosis very well, and often got a good therapeutic effect.

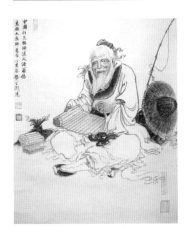

◇涪翁画像
龚学渊绘

Fuweng's portrait
Painted by Mr. GONG Xue-yuan

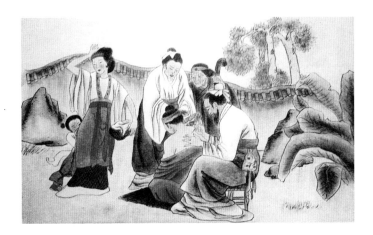

◇涪翁针刺疗疾
摄于湖南中医药大学针灸陈列馆

Fuweng was treating a patient with acupuncture
Taken in the Museum of Acupuncture and Moxibustion of Hunan University of TCM

 ## 郭玉与汉和帝

　　郭玉在民间行医时,汉和帝的贵妃小腹左边有一包块,疼痛时腹部膨胀,手足疲软,不省人事,宫中太医无能为力。于是,汉和帝令太监去请名医郭玉。郭玉到宫中后,汉和帝想考验他,亲自测试脉理,故意让手腕长得白嫩柔美的一名后宫宠臣与一位女子混杂置身在帷帐里,叫他隔着帘帏为两个"女人"诊脉。郭玉准确地判断出有一只手是男人的,后又治好了得疑难病的宫妃,汉和帝才同意他为贵妃治病。贵妃的病经郭玉诊治后,药到病除。汉和帝见郭玉确是医术高明,便将他留在宫中,封为太医院太医丞校尉。

## GUO Yu and Emperor Hedi of the Han Dynasty

During the period when GUO Yu was practicing medicine among the civilians, the imperial concubine once suffered from abdominal pain and distention with a lump on the left side. In severe attack, her pain aggravated with swollen abdomen, weakness of limbs, and even loss of consciousness. So the Emperor ordered the eunuch to invite the famous doctor GUO Yu. When GUO Yu arrived in the palace, the Emperor wanted to test him, so he let a favorite Minister of the palace who had white and delicate arms like a woman and another woman be together in the curtain, asking him to examine the pulse for two "women" across the curtain. GUO Yu accurately judged that there was a man's hand, and then cured the palace concubine of a difficult disease. The Emperor then agreed to have GUO Yu treating the imperial concubine. After receiving the treatment with medicine prescribed by Dr. GUO, the imperial concubine was cured. Then the Emperor decided that this experienced skillful Dr. GUO stayed in the palace to be an imperial physician.

# 19

## 华佗与针灸
### HUA Tuo and acupuncture-moxibustion

华佗,字元化,出生于豫州沛国谯县(今安徽亳州)的一个普通士族家庭,约生于汉冲帝永熹元年(公元 145 年),卒于汉献帝建安十三年(公元 208 年),东汉名医。

他精通内、外、妇产、小儿、针灸等各科及卫生学、药物学,尤擅长外科,被后世尊为"外科圣手""外科鼻祖"。华佗针灸治疗时,只选用一两个穴位,简单而有效。据《隋书·经籍志》记载,华佗撰有《华佗枕中灸刺经》一卷,已佚。

HUA Tuo, courtesy name Yuan Hua, was born in an ordinary scholar family in Qiao County of Pei-state of Yuzhou (currently, Bozhou City of Anhui Province), in the first year of Yongxi Age of Emperor Chong (145 A.D.) in the late stage of the Eastern Han Dynasty. He died in the 13th year of Jian'an Age of Emperor Xian of the Han Dynasty (208 A.D.), and was a well-known physician of the Eastern Han Dynasty.

Being proficient in various branches of TCM, including internal medicine, surgery, gynecology and obstetrics, pediatrics, acupuncture and moxibustion, hygiology and pharmacology, especially in surgery, HUA Tuo was named a "master of the surgery" or "the founder of Chinese surgery". In the light of book *Suishu: Jingji Zhi* (《隋书·经籍志》*History of Sui Dynasty: Records of Classics and Books*), he wrote a volume of *Huatuo Zhenzhong Jiuci Jing* (《华佗枕中灸刺经》*Classic on Moxibustion and Acupuncture by HUA Tuo*), but it was lost.

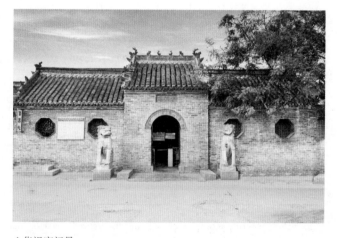

◇华祖庵门景
　位于安徽省亳州市

Outdoor scene of Ancestor HUA's Nunnery
Located in Bozhou City of Anhui Province

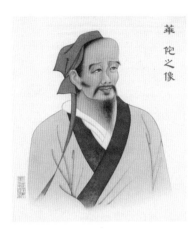

◇华佗画像
宋大仁绘

HUA Tuo's portrait
Drawn by SONG Da-ren

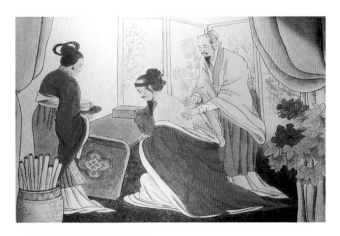

◇华佗为曹操针刺治疗头风病
摄于湖南中医药大学针灸陈列馆

HUA Tuo was treating CAO Cao's (Prime Minister of the Han Dynasty) head-wind disease with acupuncture.
Taken in the Museum of Acupuncture and Moxibustion of Hunan University of TCM

 精湛医术惹来杀身之祸

　　曹操早年患有头风病,发作时头痛难忍,请了很多医生治疗,都不见效。听说华佗医术高明,曹操就请他医治,华佗只给他扎了一针,头痛立止。曹操恐头风病再发,欲留华佗做自己的侍医。华佗禀性清高,不慕功利,执意离去。

　　不久,华佗被抓去为曹操治病。华佗诊断之后,认为曹操的病需要剖开头颅,施行手术,才能除去病根。曹操一听,勃然大怒,认为华佗要谋害他,就把华佗杀害了。华佗临死前拿出一卷医书交给狱吏,狱吏不敢接受,华佗便将书焚毁,此乃千古憾事。

## Experienced medical techniques but bring disaster

　　CAO Cao suffered from headache in his early years. During the attack he had severe pain. Though he was treated by many doctors, he failed to be treated. When he was told that HUA Tuo had skillful techniques, he asked him for treatment. Then HUA Tuo treated him by only puncturing one point with a needle, his headache stopped at once. Being afraid of having another attack of headache, CAO Cao would like to keep HUA Tuo as his own doctor. However, since HUA Tuo did not admire the utilitarianism, he refused and insisted on leaving.

　　Soon, HUA Tuo was arrested to treat CAO Cao again. After the diagnosis, he suggested that CAO Cao should receive a surgical operation on the head for treating the root cause of the disease. When CAO Cao heard it, he flew into a rage. He thought HUA Tuo wanted to kill him, so he killed HUA Tuo. Before death, HUA Tuo took out a medical book and handed it to the warder. The warder dared not accept it. HUA Tuo had to burn the book, which has been a pity for ages.

# 20

## 医圣张仲景与针药结合
## Medical sage ZHANG Zhong-jing and joint-application of acupuncture and herbal medicines

张仲景,名机,字仲景,河南南阳人,生于东汉桓帝元嘉、永兴年间(约公元 150—154 年),卒于东汉献帝建安二十四年(公元 219 年),被人尊称为医圣。

张仲景一生勤求古训,博采众方,写出了不朽的医学名著《伤寒杂病论》。书中对于针灸学的论述,有独到之处,如重药不轻针、针药并用、杂病刺法、烧针和温针刺法、阳证宜针、阴证宜灸等,反映了作者的针灸学术思想,丰富和发展了东汉以前的针灸学理论,对后世针灸学的发展也产生了深远的影响。

ZHANG Zhong-jing, i.e., ZHANG Ji (formal name), courtesy name Zhong-jing, a native from Nanyang of Henan Province, was born during Yuanjia and Yongxing ages of Emperor Heng in the Eastern Han Dynasty (150–154 A.D.), and died in the 24<sup>th</sup> year of Jian'an Age of Emperor Xian of the same dynasty (219 A.D.). He is often regarded as the medical sage of TCM.

ZHANG Zhong-jing was diligent in studying ancient mottos in his whole life and in collecting many prescriptions of various scholars, and wrote *Shanghan Zabing Lun* (《伤寒杂病论》 *Treatise on Febrile and Miscellaneous Diseases*), an immortal medical masterpiece of TCM. In this book, his viewpoints on acupuncture and moxibustion were unique and profound, for instance, putting stress on acupuncture and herbal medicines equally by joint application of them, adopting reasonable needling techniques for miscellaneous diseases, performing hot-red needle or warm needle, employing acupuncture to treat yang syndrome, and performing moxibustion to treat yin syndrome,

◇《仲景全书》中针灸内容

明万历刻本,中国中医科学院图书馆藏

The contents on acupuncture and moxibustion in *Zhongjing Quanshu* (《仲景全书》 *Zhongjing's Complete Collection*) Block-printed edition of Wanli Age of the Ming Dynasty, collected by the Library of CACMS etc. All of these greatly enrich and renew the related theories established before the Eastern Han Dynasty, and produce a far-reaching influence on the development of acupuncture-moxibustion medicine in the later generations.

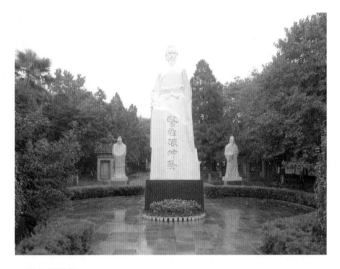

◇张仲景雕塑
　摄于河南省南阳医圣祠

ZHANG Zhong-jing's statue
Photographed in Nanyang Medical Sage Temple of Henan Province

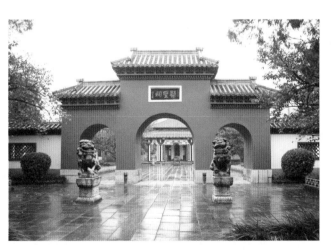

◇医圣祠门景
　摄于河南省南阳医圣祠

Outdoor scene of Nanyang Medical Sage Temple
Photographed in Nanyang Medical Sage Temple of Henan Province

##  张仲景与《伤寒杂病论》

东汉建安以来，由于伤寒的流行，仅十年间，张仲景原先超过200人的家族中，三分之二的亲属都染病去世。痛心之余，张仲景精研医术，收集当时的部分重要医书，撰成《伤寒杂病论》，该书后世重新编辑为《伤寒论》与《金匮要略》两书。

《伤寒杂病论》最重要的贡献是奠定了中医学辨证论治的基础，其中的方剂组方精炼，配伍严谨，疗效精奇，被后世称之为"经方"。该书成为后世学习中医学的必修经典，张仲景也被尊之为"医圣"。

## ZHANG Zhong-jing and Shanghan Zabing Lun

Since Jian'an in the Eastern Han Dynasty, due to the epidemic febrile diseases, two-thirds of over 200 relatives from ZHANG Zhong-jing's families died of illness within 10 years. In spite of being distressed, he studied medicine hard by collecting some important medical books at that time and compiled *Shanghan Zabing Lun*, which was later re-edited into two books: *Shanghan Lun* (《伤寒论》*Treatise on Febrile Diseases*) and *Jingui Yaolue* (《金匮要略》*Synopsis of the Golden Chamber*).

The most important contribution of *Shanghan Zabing Lun* is to lay the foundation of TCM syndrome differentiation and treatment of diseases. The prescriptions recorded are refined with strict combinations and remarkable effects, which are called "classical formulae" by later generations. This book has become a compulsory classic for students to learn Chinese medicine. ZHANG Zhong-jing has also been honored as "the medical sage".

# 21

## 皇甫谧与《针灸甲乙经》
## HUANGFU Mi and *Zhenjiu Jiayi Jing* (*The A-B Classic of Acupuncture and Moxibustion*)

皇甫谧,幼名静,字士安,自号玄晏先生,安定朝那(今甘肃灵台县朝那镇)人,生于东汉献帝建安二十年(公元215年),卒于西晋武帝太康三年(公元282年)。

皇甫谧是魏晋之际一位博学多才的文学家、历史学家和医学家,一生著作丰富,针灸学方面著有《黄帝三部针灸甲乙经》,简称《针灸甲乙经》或《甲乙经》,系将《灵枢》《素问》《黄帝明堂经》类编而成,全书共12卷,128篇。该书是我国现存最早的针灸专著,集晋代以前针灸学之大成,是继《内经》《难经》之后针灸学的又一次总结,在针灸发展史上起了承先启后的作用。后世一些著名的针灸著作,基本上都是在《甲乙经》的基础上发挥而成的。

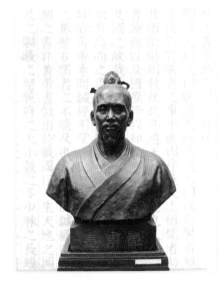

◇皇甫谧雕塑
　中国中医科学院针灸研究所针灸博物馆藏
HUANGFU Mi's statue
Collected by Chinese Museum of Acupuncture and Moxibustion, CACMS

HUANGFU Mi, HUANGFU Jing in his childhood name, courtesy name Shi'an and self-called Mr. Xuanyan, a native of Chaona Township of An'ding (currently, Lingtai County of Gansu Province), was born in the 20<sup>th</sup> year of Jian'an Age of the Eastern Han Dynasty (215 A.D.), and died in the 3<sup>rd</sup> year of Taikang Age of Emperor Wu in the Western Jin Dynasty (282 A.D.).

HUANGFU Mi was an erudite and versatile writer, historian and medical scientist. He wrote many medical books as *Zhenjiu Jiayi Jing* (《针灸甲乙经》*The A-B Classic of Acupuncture and Moxibustion*), *Huangdi Sanbu Zhenjiu Jiayi Jing* (《黄帝三部针灸甲乙经》*Three Collections of the Yellow Emperor's A-B Classic of Acupuncture and Moxibustion*) in full name or *Jiayi Jing* in short, which is composed of *Lingshu* and *Suwen* of *the Huangdi Neijing*, and *Huangdi Mingtang Jing*, containing 12 volumes and 128 chapters. It is the extant earliest monograph on acupuncture and moxibustion, and a complete collection of the related learnings accumulated before the Jin Dynasty. It is another summary on acupuncture and moxibustion after *Huangdi Neijing* and *Nanjing*, playing an important role in linking the past and the future. The later generations' well-known works on acupuncture and moxibustion are basically developed on the basis of *Zhenjiu Jiayi Jing*.

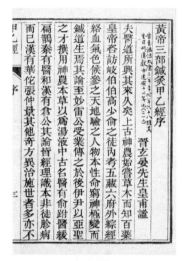

◇《针灸甲乙经》书影

明万历刻《古今医统正脉全书》本，中国中医科学院图书馆藏

Photocopy of *Zhenjiu Jiayi Jing*
Block-printed version of *Gujin Yitong Zhengmai Quanshu* (《古今医统正脉全书》*A Complete Collection of the Orthodox Medical Works*) from Wanli Age of the Ming Dynasty, collected by the Library of CACMS

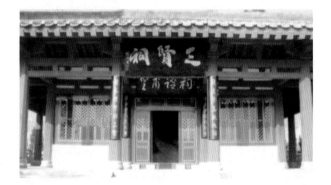

◇皇甫谧祠

位于甘肃省灵台县城荆山

The Memorial Temple of HUANGFU Mi
Located at Jingshan of Lingtai County of Gansu Province

# 22

# 葛洪与女灸法家鲍姑
## GE Hong and BAO Gu (a female moxibustion practitioner)

　　葛洪,字稚川,号抱朴子,道号葛仙翁,丹阳句容(今江苏省句容市)人,约生于晋太康二年(公元281年),卒于咸康七年(公元341年),东晋著名道学家和医学家。葛洪精通医术与炼丹术,所撰《肘后备急方》主要记述各种急症的治疗方法,采用灸法甚多,特别是将灸法广泛运用于各类疾病的治疗中,对灸法治病的效用、操作、宜忌等均作了较全面的论述,是记载灸疗较早较多的古代医学文献之一。

　　鲍姑,葛洪之妻,名潜光(约公元309—363年),山西长治人,是我国医学史上第一位女性灸疗家。鲍姑医术精良,擅长灸法,以艾线灸治赘瘤和赘疣而闻名于世。她长期与丈夫葛洪在广州罗浮山炼丹行医,岭南人民尊称她为"鲍仙姑"。遗憾的是,鲍姑没有留下什么著作,后人认为,她的灸疗经验可能渗入到葛洪的《肘后备急方》中。

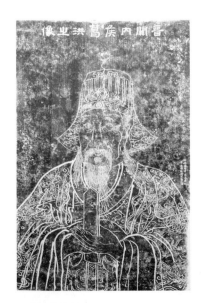

◇葛洪像碑拓
　　摄于上海中医药博物馆

Rubbings of GE Hong's portrait stele
Taken in Shanghai Museum of Chinese Medicine

　　GE Hong, courtesy name Zhichuan, and assumed name Baopuzi: and also called GE Xian-weng in Taoism name, was a famous Taoist and medical expert from Jurong of Danyang (currently, Jurong City of Jiangsu Province). He was born in about the 2<sup>nd</sup> year of Taikang Age of the Jin Dynasty (281 A.D.) and died in the 7<sup>th</sup> year of Xiankang Age of the Eastern Jin Dynasty (341 A.D.). GE Hong was very proficient in medical skills and spagirism. He wrote *Zhouhou Beiji Fang* (《肘后备急方》*Handbook of Prescriptions for Emergencies*) to record a lot of therapeutic methods for various emergencies, with moxibustion widely applied in the treatment. In this book, he made a comprehensive exposition on the efficacy, operation, indications and contraindications of moxibustion therapy. It is one of the earlier ancient medical documents on moxibustion therapy.

BAO Gu, GE Hong's wife, called Qian-guang (309–363 A.D.), was from Changzhi City of Shanxi Province. She was the first female moxibustion practitioner in Chinese medical history. Being highly qualified in medical skills particularly in moxibustion therapy, she was well-known for treating neoplasma and excrescence with moxa-floss. She and her husband performed spagirism and medicine in Luofushan region of Guangzhou for a long time. People in Lingnan (Current Guangdong Province and Guangxi Zhuang Atonomous Region) region respected her and called her as "Bao Xian-gu" (Xiangu means female immortal). But unfortunately, she didn't leave any works. It was thought by the descendants that her experience on moxibustion might have been included in GE Hong's book *Zhouhou Beiji Fang*.

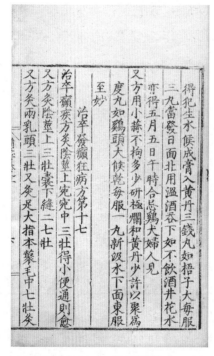

◇《肘后备急方》书影
明万历刻本,中国中医科学院图书馆藏

Photocopy of *Zhouhou Beiji Fang*
Block-printed edition of Wanli Age of the Ming Dynasty; kept in the Library of CACMS

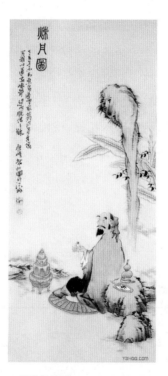

◇葛洪炼丹图
康峰绘

GE Hong was concocting magic pills
Painted by KANG Feng

# 23
# 南北朝徐氏家族针灸派系
## XU's family acupuncture-moxibustion faction during the Northern and Southern dynasties

南北朝时,以医学立业的徐氏家族,自创始人徐熙始,父子兄弟家世相传七代,出现了徐熙、徐秋夫、徐道度、徐文伯、徐嗣伯、徐之才等 12 位名医,成为我国较大的家族针灸派系。他们均精通医术,在当时享有较高的声誉,在我国医学发展史上占有一席之地。其中,在针灸方面最为有名的是徐秋夫与徐文伯两位,史书上记载了较多关于他们针灸治疗疾病的故事,广为人知的是"徐秋夫针刺疗鬼"和"徐文伯泻三阴交下胎"。

During the Northern and Southern Dynasties, XU's clan had a respectable medical career and handed it down successively for 7 generations beginning from XU Xi. A total of 12 well-known physicians as XU Xi, XU Qiu-fu, XU Dao-du, XU Wen-bo, XU Si-bo, XU Zhi-cai, et al appeared and formed a big acupuncture-moxibustion family faction. Well mastering medical skills, they all enjoyed a higher reputation and took an important position in the development of Chinese medical history. Among them, the most well-known members are XU Qiu-fu and XU Wen-bo, and quite a lot of stories about their acupuncture treatment of disorders had been recorded. The extensively known stories are: "XU Qiu-fu treated evils successfully with acupuncture" and "XU Wen-bo performed reducing-needling manipulation at Sanyinjiao (SP 6) to induce abortion".

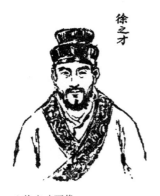

◇徐之才画像

**XU Zhi-cai' portrait**

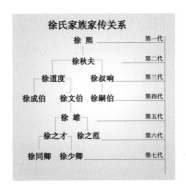

◇徐氏家族家传关系

**XU's family tree**

# 24

# 针灸学传入朝鲜、日本
# Introduction of acupuncture-moxibustion to North Korea and Japan

汉以前,由于交通等方面的原因,国内外医学交流还比较少。三国两晋南北朝时期,随着陆上、海上交通的逐渐发达,中外交往亦渐频繁,其间自然也带来了医药卫生方面的交往。

早在公元 6 世纪针灸学就传到邻近国家,此时期中国针灸专著《针灸甲乙经》传入朝鲜。公元 514 年,针灸术传到朝鲜;公元 550 年,灸治术传到日本;公元 552 年,我国以《针经》赠日本钦明天皇;公元 561 年(南陈文帝天嘉二年),吴(今苏州吴中区一带)人知聪携带《神农本草经》《脉经》《明堂图》等共 164 卷,经由高句丽(知聪在此居留 1 年)赴日本传授中国医学,对朝鲜、日本的医学,产生了重要影响。

Before the Han Dynasty, due to traffic and other reasons, domestic and foreign medical exchanges were relatively few. In the periods of Three Kingdoms, the Western and Eastern Jin Dynasties, and the Southern and Northern Dynasties, along with the development of the overland traffic and marine traffic, the Chinese and foreign exchanges became more frequent gradually, meanwhile, brining about medical and health exchanges.

As early as the 6th century, acupuncture and moxibustion were introduced to the neighboring countries, when, *Zhenjiu Jiayi Jing*, a monograph on acupuncture and moxibustion, was introduced to North Korea. In 514 A.D., acupuncture and moxibustion techniques were spread to North Korea. In 550, the moxibustion therapy was introduced to Japan. In 552 A.D., Chinese government presented *Zhenjing* to Emperor Kimmei of Japan. In the 2nd year of Tianjia Age of Emperor CHEN Wen-di of Nan Dynasty (561 A.D.), Zhi Cong (a monk) from Wu (current Wuzhong district of Suzhou) took 164 volumes of medical books including *Shennong Bencao Jing* (《神农本草经》 *Shennong's Classic of Materia Medica*), *Maijing* (《脉经》 *Pulse Classic*), *Mingtang Tu* (《明堂图》 *Chart of Acupoints*), etc. to Japan to impart Chinese medicine by way of Gaojuli (where he stayed for one year), giving rise to a great impact on the traditional medicine of North Korea and Japan.

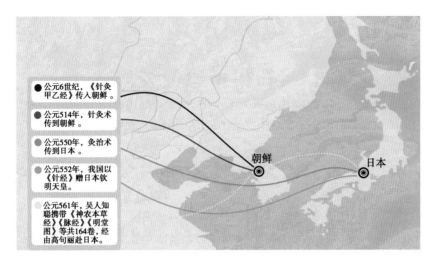

◇针灸传入朝鲜、日本线路图

Routes of spread of acupuncture-moxibustion to North Korea and Japan

敦煌卷子《灸法图》《新集备急灸经》
*Illustrations of Moxibustion and New Collection of Moxibustion Classic for Emergencies* in Dunhuang's incomplete manuscripts

# 25

# 敦煌卷子《灸法图》《新集备急灸经》
## *Illustrations of Moxibustion and New Collection of Moxibustion Classic for Emergencies* in Dunhuang's incomplete manuscripts

1900 年，甘肃省敦煌县莫高窟藏经洞发掘出唐人写绘的《灸法图》《新集备急灸经》残卷，今分别藏于英国伦敦图书馆与法国国家图书馆。《灸法图》各卷绘有人体正（或背）面的灸穴图像，分段论述各类病症的名称、主治、所灸腧穴及其壮数，图文对照，是我国现存最早、有绘图的灸疗专著。《新集备急灸经》残卷有甲乙两个版本，甲本载此书小序、人体上半身穴位图、正文（某某病证，取某某腧穴，壮数）以及人神禁忌内容，乙本仅有人神禁忌，无图。与传世针灸古籍相比，这两部敦煌灸法文献对病证及所灸腧穴的记载有所差异，对考察古代灸疗取穴、腧穴命名演变等提供了珍贵资料，有很高的学术和史料价值。同时，也反映出隋唐前后对艾灸疗法的重视与广泛运用。

In 1900, some incomplete manuscripts of *Jiufa Tu* (《灸法图》*Illustrations of Moxibustion*) and *Xinji Beiji Jiujing* (《新集备急灸经》*New Collection of Moxibustion Classic for Emergencies*) written and drawn by scholars of the Tang Dynasty were excavated from the Mogao Grottoes of Dunhuang County, Gansu Province, which are now preserved respectively in the London Library (Britain) and the National Library of France (Bibliothèque nationale de France). In each volume of *Jiufa Tu*, there were some drawn pictures of human body with moxa points either on the front side or the back side, and corresponding legends to describe the names of various conditions, symptoms or illnesses, acupoint formulas and number of moxa-cones applied. It is the earliest extant monography of moxibustion with illustrations and annotations in China. The incomplete manuscripts of *Xinji Beiji Jiujing* have two versions, A and B. In version A, there are a brief preface of the whole book, upper human-body pictures with acupoints, main text (name of illnesses, selected acupoints, and number of moxa-cones applied), and taboos for human and Gods. While in version B, only taboos for human and Gods were recorded, without any illustrations. Compared with the handed down ancient books on acupuncture-moxibustion, some related contents about the clinical conditions and acupoints selected in these two sets of literature excavated from the Mogao Grottoes have some differences, but provide

敦煌卷子《灸法图》《新集备急灸经》

*Illustrations of Moxibustion and New Collection of Moxibustion Classic for Emergencies* in Dunhuang's incomplete manuscripts

rather valuable materials for investigating the evolution of acupoint-selection for moxibustion and nomenclature of acupoints in the ancient times. They have quite high academic and historical data values, also reflecting the importance and extensive application of moxibustion therapy about in the periods of the Sui and Tang dynasties.

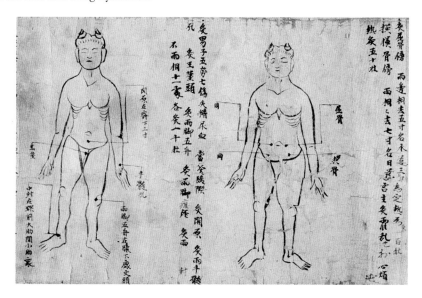

◇敦煌卷子《灸法图》
　英国伦敦图书馆藏

Dunhuang's incomplete manuscripts of *Jiufa Tu*
Kept in London Library in Britain

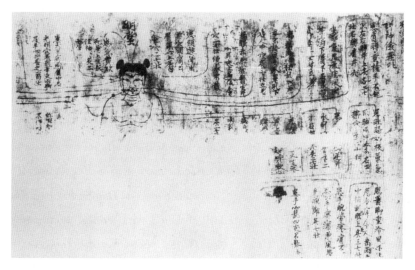

◇敦煌卷子《新集备急灸经》
　法国国家图书馆藏

Dunhuang's incomplete manuscripts *of Xinji Beiji Jiujing*
Kept in the National Library of France (Bibliothèque nationale de France)

# 26

# 唐代针灸名医甄权
ZHEN Quan, a famous acupuncturist of the Tang Dynasty

甄权,许州扶沟人(今河南扶沟县),约出生于南北朝时期西魏大同六年(公元540年),卒于唐贞观十七年(公元643年),隋唐年间著名针灸医家。

甄权针术高明,临床取穴不多,却效如桴鼓。同时,他亦谙养生,获103岁高龄。唐太宗曾亲临其家咨询药性,视其饮食,赐以衣服几杖,并授其"朝散大夫"之号。他著有《针经钞》《明堂人形图》《针方》及《脉经》,均已佚,但其部分内容尚可见于《千金方》《外台秘要》等书,对后世有一定影响。

ZHEN Quan, a native of Fugou of Xuzhou (currently, Fugou County of Henan Province), was born in the 6th year of Datong Age of the Western Wei Kingdom during the Southern and Northern Dynasties (540 A.D.), and died in the 17th year of Zhenguan Age of the Tang Dynasty (643 A.D.). He was a famous acupuncturist in the period of the Sui and Tang Dynasties.

ZHEN Quan was very skillful in acupuncture techniques. When practicing acupuncture, he selected fewer acupoints in every session of treatment, but often obtained a good therapeutic effect. He also knew well about health preservation, and thus lived for 103 years. Emperor Taizong (the second emperor of the Tang Dynasty) himself once visited ZHEN's home to consult him about the properties of many materia medica, and to inquire his diet, granted him clothes and walking stick, and awarded him a title of "Chao San Dafu" (high-class medical official without actual authority). ZHEN wrote *Zhenjing Chao* (《针经钞》*Transcribed Passages from the Classic of Acupuncture*), *Mingtang Renxing Tu* (《明堂人形图》*Chart of Acupoints Shown on Human Figure*), *Zhenfang* (《针方》*Acupuncture Prescriptions*) and *Maijing*, but all of them have been lost. Fortunately some of the contents can be found in *Qianjin Fang* (《千金方》*Prescriptions Worth a Thousand Gold*), *Waitai Miyao* and some other books, which influence the later ages.

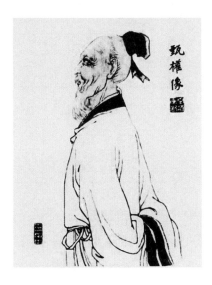

◇甄权画像

引自《中国历代名医图传》（陈雪楼主编，江苏科学技术出版社，1987年）

ZHEN Quan's portrait
Cited from book *Zhongguo Lidai Mingyi Tuzhuan* (《中国历代名医图传》*The Photographic Biography of Chinese Famous Physicians of the Successive Dynasties*) (Editor-in-chief CHEN Xue-lou, published by Jiangsu Science and Technology Press in 1987)

 甄权医案

　　《旧唐书·甄权传》记载，唐代鲁州刺史库狄嵚练习射箭时扭伤了肩部，不能挽弓。他找了很多名医治疗，都不见效，最后找到了甄权。甄权治病很有特色，他治疗时所选穴位和前几位名医完全一样，不同之处在于，针刺治疗时，要求患者保持原来射箭的姿势，结果一扎针，库狄嵚的肩痛就好了。

## A medical case of ZHEN Quan

　　The story is found in the book *Jiutangshu: Zhenquan Zhuan* (《旧唐书·甄权传》*History of the Late Han Dynasty: ZHEN Quan's Biography*): KU Di-qin, a state official of Luzhou in the Tang Dynasty sprained his shoulder during archery exercise and could not draw the bow. He received treatment from many famous doctors but he still failed to be treated, and finally he came to ZHEN Quan. ZHEN Quan's technique was unique. Though the points selected were completely the same as those used by the previous physicians, the way of treatment was rather different. While puncturing the points with needles, ZHEN Quan asked the patient to keep the original archery posture. As a result, KU's shoulder pain was relieved at once after being punctured with needles.

# 27

# 杨上善与《太素》
## YANG Shang-shan and *Taisu* (*Great Simplicity*)

杨上善,隋唐时期著名医家(约公元 575—670 年),隋大业年间任太医侍御。

杨上善撰有《黄帝内经太素》(简称《太素》)30 卷。该书系取《素问》及《灵枢》内容重新编次加以注解而成,保存了《内经》中一些原文的较早面貌,是《内经》的早期传本之一,亦是现存最早注释《内经》的专著,为研读《内经》提供了极为珍贵的医学资料。他还著有《黄帝内经明堂》,今仅存残本第一卷,是对中国第一部腧穴经典——《黄帝明堂经》的重新注解与编撰,具有很高的文献价值。

YANG Shang-shan, a famous medical specialist during the Sui and Tang Dynasties (about 575–670 A.D.), was appointed to be an imperial physician serving the emperor in Daye Age of the Sui Dynasty.

He wrote a book *Huangdi Neijing Taisu* (《黄帝内经太素》*Grand Simplicity of The Yellow Emperor's Inner Classic*), simplied as *Taisu* (《太素》*Great Simplicity*), with 30 volumes in which he recompiled the contents of *Suwen* and *Lingshu* of *Huangdi Neijing*, and made a detailed annotation. This book preserves the earlier content of the original text of *Huangdi Neijing*, is one of the earlier inherited versions of *Huangdi Neijing*, and is also the extant earliest monograph on the annotated *Huangdi Neijing*. It provides a very precious medical data for extensively studying *Neijing*. In addition, he also wrote book *Huangdi Neijing Mingtang* (《黄帝内经明堂》*The Yellow Emperor's Inner Classic of Acupoints*), but only its first volume (incomplete) is preserved nowadays. It is a re-annotation and re-compilation of Chinese first classical book on acupoints (*Huangdi Mingtang Jing*), processing very high literature value.

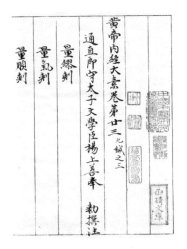

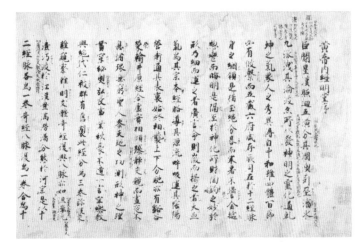

◇《黄帝内经太素》书影
日本抄本，中国中医科学院图书馆藏

Photocopy of *Huangdi Neijing Taisu*
The Japanese transcript, preserved by
the Library of CACMS

◇《黄帝内经明堂》书影
日本尊经阁文库写本

Photocopy of *Huangdi Neijing Mingtang*
Hand-copied book of Japanese Sonkeikaku Library

##  《黄帝内经太素》的流传

　　《太素》于唐中期传入日本，孝谦天皇发布敕令，《太素》为首选必读医书，后该书在中国及日本均遭亡佚。19世纪20年代，在日本仁和寺发现《太素》卷子抄本，引起了学术界较大震动。此后，我国近世通儒杨守敬（字惺吾）先生访日时将《太素》的影抄本携带回国。后由清代学者袁昶主持刊刻《太素》，对《太素》的广泛流传起到了积极的推动作用。又经清人萧延平校勘，质量与内容均较精良，后经人民卫生出版社影印重刊，影响较大。《太素》的重新发现，对于推动《内经》学术研究具有重要的意义。

## The Spread of Huangdi Neijing Taisu

　　*Taisu* was introduced into Japan in the mid-Tang Dynasty. Emperor Xiao Qian issued an edict that the book should be a must-read medical book. And later, the book was lost in China and Japan. In the 1920s, a transcript of *Taisu* was found in the Ren He Temple in Japan, which caused a shock in the academic circles. Later, Mr. YANG Shou-jing, a contemporary scholar in China, brought back a copy of *Taisu* after his visit to Japan and YUAN Chang, a scholar in the Qing Dynasty, presided over the publication and engraving of *Taisu*, which played a positive role in promoting the wide spread of the book. After collation by XIAO Yan-ping of the Qing Dynasty, the book had been improved in quality and content, and then reprinted by the People's Health Publishing House. The rediscovery of *Taisu* is of great significance in promoting the academic research on *Huangdi Neijing*.

# 28

# 药王孙思邈与针灸
SUN Si-miao (King of Medicine) and acupuncture-moxibustion

孙思邈,隋唐时京兆华原(今陕西省铜川市耀州区)人,约生于隋文帝开皇元年(公元581年),卒于唐高宗永淳元年(公元682年),人称"孙真人",唐代杰出的医药学家。

孙思邈通晓临床各科,撰有《备急千金要方》及《千金翼方》各30卷。该书集唐代以前医药学之大成,被誉为我国最早的一部临床医学百科全书,其中针灸学内容非常丰富,主张针、灸、药结合应用。书中还记载了"阿是穴"的针刺取穴方法,绘制了彩色"明堂三人图"等,推动了针灸学的发展。

SUN Si-miao, courtesy name "SUN Zhen-ren" (an immortal term in Taoism), a native of Huayuan (currently, Yaozhou district in Tongchuan City of Shaanxi Province) of the capital district in the period of the Sui and Tang Dynasties, was born in about the first year of Kaihuang Age of Emperor Wendi of the Sui Dynasty (581 A.D.) and died in the first year of Yongchun Age of Emperor Gaozong in the Tang Dynasty (682 A.D.). He was an outstanding medical specialist.

SUN Si-miao was proficient in every subject of clinical medicine, and wrote *Beiji Qianjin Yaofang* (《备急千金要方》*Important Prescriptions Worth a Thousand Gold for Emergencies*) and *Qianjin Yifang* (《千金翼方》*A Supplement to the Essential Prescriptions Worth a Thousand Gold*) with 30 volumes respectively. The former book contains a great deal of achievements in Chinese medicine prior to the Tang Dynasty, has an extraordinary rich content about acupuncture and moxibustion learnings, and advocates joint application of acupuncture, moxibustion and medicinal herbs. It is honored to be the earliest encyclopedia of clinical medicine in China, in which some methods for needling "Ashi-point" were recorded and a color "picture of three human figures with acupoints" was drawn up. SUN Si-miao made a great contribution to the development of acupuncture-moxibustion medicine.

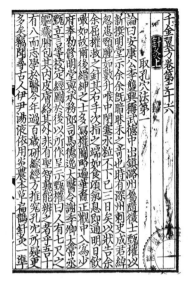

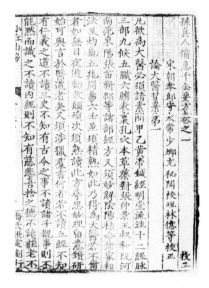

◇《千金翼方》书影

清光绪四年影元刻本，中国医学科学院图书馆藏

Photocopy of *Qianjin Yifang*
Block-printed edition of the 4th year of Emperor Guangxu Age of the Qing Dynasty, copied according to the Yuan Dynasty's edition, collected by the Library of CACMS

◇《备急千金要方》书影

元刻本，中国中医科学院图书馆藏

Photocopy of *Beiji Qianjin Yaofang*
Block-printed edition of the Yuan Dynasty, collected by the Library of CACMS

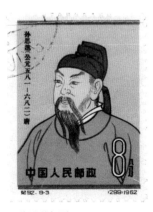

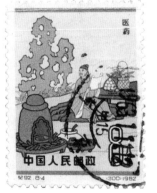

◇孙思邈邮票

中国古代科学家邮票，1962年12月1日影印版，周建杨教授藏

Stamps for memorizing SUN Si-miao
Stamps for memorizing Chinese ancient scientists, photographic edition issued on December 1, 1962, collected by Prof. ZHOU Jian-yang

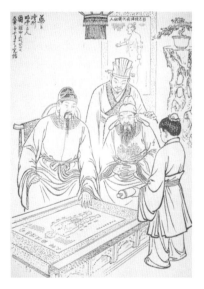

◇孙思邈彩绘明堂图

摄于陕西省耀县药王山孙思邈展室

Colored human figure of acupoints painted by SUN Si-miao
Taken in the exhibition room of SUN Si-miao, the Medicine-king Mountain, at Yao County of Shaanxi Province

### 孙思邈妙解阴阳

孙思邈以毕生的智慧,精研医学和百家学说,到百岁时,已是经验丰富,炉火纯青,形成了一套精辟的医学理论。他认为,大自然有四时五行,寒暑交替,有其变化的规律。人体和自然界同是一理。人体生理有五脏六腑,呼吸吐纳,精气往常,也有其自身的规律。如果阴阳失调,就会导致疾病。医生的职责就是调节和把握人体阴阳平衡,以达到治病的目的。他说,"良医导之以药石,救之以针剂,圣人和之以至德,辅之以人事。故形体有可愈之疾,天地有可消之灾"。他不相信鬼、神、天,反对宿命论,相信人只要善于"妙解"和调理,就会防止疾病的发生。他的这些理论是中国古代医学史上全新的科学理论。

## Excellent interpretation of yin-yang by SUN Si-miao

With lifelong wisdom, SUN Si-miao elaborately studied medicine and learned various schools of thought. By the time he was a hundred years old, he had already experienced and had formed a profound set of medical theories. He believed that nature has four seasons and five elements, alternating with cold and heat regularly, following the natural laws. The human body is the same as nature, which has five Zang and six Fu organs, breathing by inhaling and exhaling with vital qi circulating regularly, following the body's own patterns. Imbalance of yin and yang will lead to diseases. The duty of a physician is to regulate and keep the balance of yin-yang of the body for treatment of diseases. He said, "The good physician treats diseases with medicine, save patients with needles; the saint harmonizes with virtue and is able to choose right personnel to run a country. Therefore, the illness of body can be treated, disaster in nature eliminated." Being against fatalism, he did not believe in ghosts and Gods. He thought that as long as people were able to have a "good interpretation" and self-regulation, the occurrence of diseases would be prevented. These theories are entirely new scientific theories in the history of ancient Chinese medicine.

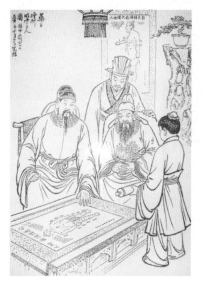

◇孙思邈彩绘明堂图
**摄于陕西省耀县药王山孙思邈展室**

Colored human figure of acupoints painted by SUN Si-miao
Taken in the exhibition room of SUN Si-miao, the Medicine-king Mountain, at Yao County of Shaanxi Province

# 29

## 官方最早的针灸教育专科

## The earliest official specialized subject on the education of acupuncture and moxibustion

古代的针灸教育，主要是师徒传授和家世相传的民间教育，大约到了公元 5 世纪末，才有了官办的医学教育。公元 624 年，唐政府在京都长安设立太医署，这是一所规模相当大的官办医学院校，可视为中央医科大学，其医学教育分为 4 科：医科、针科、按摩科和咒禁科，这是首次在古代官方教育中出现了针灸专门学科。《唐书·职官志》载有唐太医署设针科的情况，"针博士一人，针助教一人，针师十人，针工二十人，针生二十人"。

In the ancient times, Chinese education on acupuncture and moxibustion was mainly realized by way of folk teacher-apprentice model and father-son handed down model. Official medical education had not appeared until the end of the 5th century. In 624 A.D., the government of Tang Dynasty set up an Imperial Physician Medical Academy in its capital Chang'an. The medical academy is in fact a big official medical college, similar to a current central medical university. Its medical education includes 4 subjects: medicine, acupuncture, massage and incantation-prohibition. It is the first time that acupuncture as a special discipline appeared in the ancient official education. In book *Tangshu: Zhiguan Zhi* (《唐书·职官志》*The History of Tang Dynasty: Records of Posts and Officials*), it is recorded that "One erudite for acupuncture, one teaching assistant on acupuncture, 10 acupuncturists, 20 junior acupuncture assistants and 20 students for acupuncture", displaying the status of the set acupuncture discipline in the Imperial Medical Academy of the Tang Dynasty.

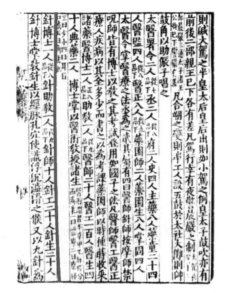

◇唐太医署设针科

　引自《唐书·职官志》

Acupuncture subject was set up in the Imperial Medical Academy in the Tang Dynasty

Quoted from book *Tangshu: Zhiguan Zhi*

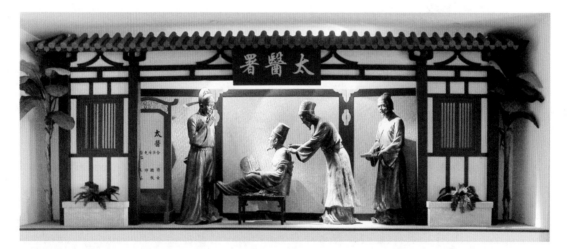

◇唐太医署复原场景

　摄于上海中医药博物馆

The scene of the reverted Imperial Medical Academy of the Tang Dynasty

Taken in the Shanghai Museum of TCM

# 30

## 王焘与《外台秘要》

## WANG Tao and *Waitai Miyao* (*Secret Remedies from the Imperial Library*)

王焘，唐时郿县（今陕西省眉县）人，约出生于唐总章三年（公元670年），卒于唐天宝十四年（公元755年），唐代著名医学家。

王焘遍访名医，掌握了大量医学知识，造诣很深，撰成《外台秘要》40卷。书中汇集有唐以前众多医家的灸疗资料，关于艾柱的大小、灸量作了详细规定，对于灸法的补泻问题，在理论上作了较深刻的阐述，是研究灸法的重要文献。王焘还十分重视经脉腧穴的相对位置关系，将十二经脉分别绘成十二人形图，即十二彩色明堂图，图中用不同颜色标出十二经脉。

WANG Tao, a native of the Mei County (currently, Mei County of Shaanxi Province), a notable medical specialist of the Tang Dynasty, was born in about the 3$^{rd}$ year of the Zongzhang Age (670 A.D.) and died in the 14$^{th}$ year of Tianbao Age (755 A.D.).

WANG Tao visited many well-known medical specialists, learned a great deal of medical knowledge and was very accomplished. He wrote a book *Waitai Miyao* (《外台秘要》*Secret Remedies from the Imperial Library*) with 40 volumes which contains abundant data about moxibustion therapy from many medical experts before the Tang Dynasty. In this book, he made a detailed stipulation about the size of moxa cone, dosage for each treatment, reinforcing and reducing methods of moxibustion. He also made rather far-reaching explanations about the theory, so it is an essential document in the

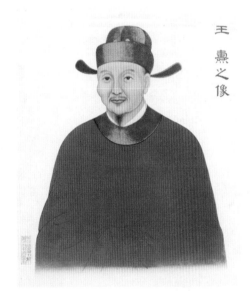

◇王焘画像
宋大仁绘

WANG Tao's portrait
Drawn by SONG Da-ren

research of moxibustion therapy. Additionally, he thought highly of the relative position-correlation between the meridian and the acupoint, drew up color charts of 12 regular meridians on 12 human figures respectively, that was known as 12 colored *Ming Tang Tu (Chart of Acupoints)*, with each regular meridian marked with different colors.

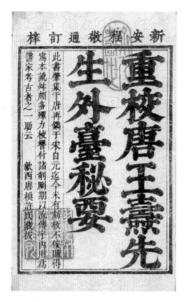

◇《外台秘要》书影
　明刻本，中国中医科学院图书馆藏

Photocopy of *Waitai Miyao*
Block-printed edition of the Ming Dynasty, collected by the Library of CACMS

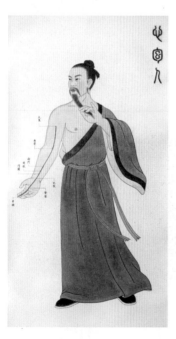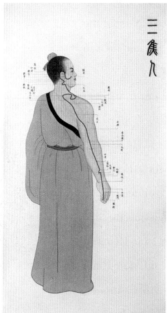

◇《外台秘要》心包人形图，三焦人形图
　青岛孙永显，1992 年重绘

Human figure of the Pericardium Meridian and human figure of the Three Triple Burner Meridian in book *Waitai Miyao*
Redrew by SUN Yong-xian from Qingdao in 1992

# 31

## 鉴真东渡日本传授针灸

## Monk Jianzhen's voyaging eastward to Japan to pass on acupuncture and moxibustion

鉴真(公元 688—763 年),姓淳于,江苏扬州人,精于佛典和医药。他受日本的邀请赴日传授佛学和医学,率弟子数十人,先后 6 次渡海,跨时 11 年,于公元 754 年到达日本首都。

鉴真通晓医学,精通本草,他把我国中药鉴别、炮制、配方、收藏、应用等技术带到了日本,并传授医学,热忱为患者治病,为中日两国人民友好和两国文化、医药交流做出了巨大贡献,人称为汉方医药始祖,日本之神农。鉴真大师东渡日本时,携带《黄帝内经太素》等医学著作与诸多药物,向日本人传授经络腧穴及针灸方法,并介绍了人体经穴图,极大地促进了日本中医药和针灸学的发展。

Jianzhen (688–763 A.D.), CHUNYU in surname, a native of Yangzhou of Jiangsu Province, was proficient in Buddhist philosophy and Chinese medicine. He was invited by Japan to teach Buddnism and medicine. He once led dozens of disciples and tried six times in crossing East China Sea, on which he spent 11 years, and finally arrived at Japanese Capital Nara successfully in 754 A.D.

Monk Jianzhen was very well-versed in medicine and materia medica. He took a variety of Chinese techniques about the identification, processing, magistral formulae, store and application of Chinese materia medica to Japan. He also passed on Chinese medicine to Japanese people, and enthusiastically treated diseases for them. He made a great contribution to Sino-Japanese people's friendship, cultural and medical exchanges, and was revered as "the founder of Japanese TCM" and

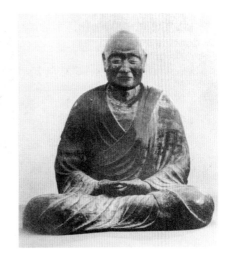

◇鉴真像

摄于中国国家博物馆

Monk Jianzhen's portrait

Taken in National Museum of China

"Japanese Shennong" by Japanese people. When voyaging eastward to Japan, Monk Jianzhen also took some medical works including *Huangdi Neijing Taisu*, and a lot of herbal medicines to Japan. He introduced meridians, acupoints, and acupuncture techniques to Japanese friends, and taught them the human diagrams of acupoints, greatly promoting the development of Japanese acupuncture-moxibustion and Chinese medicine.

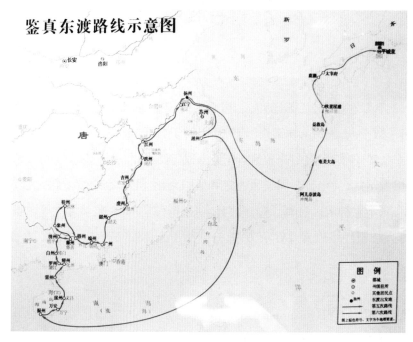

◇鉴真东渡路线示意图
摄于中国国家博物馆

Sketch map showing Monk Jianzhen's voyaging eastward to Japan
Taken in National Museum of China

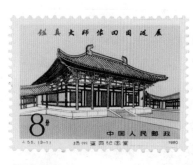
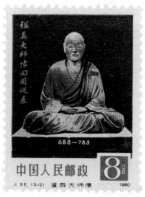
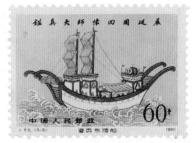

◇鉴真邮票
1980 年发行,周建杨教授藏

Stamps for memorizing Monk Jianzhen
Issued in 1980, collected by Prof. ZHOU Jian-yang

## 矢志不渝 6 次东渡的鉴真大师

唐开元二十一年（公元 733 年），日本遣僧人荣睿、普照随遣唐使来我国留学，并邀请高僧赴日弘法授戒。天宝元年（公元 742 年），鉴真接受日本僧人邀请。天宝二年（公元 743 年），鉴真和他的弟子祥彦、道兴等开始东渡。10 年之内 5 次渡海，历尽艰险，均未成功。第 5 次东渡失败后，62 岁的鉴真大师双目失明，他的大弟子祥彦圆寂，邀请他的日本僧人也病故了，但他东渡宏愿始终不移。唐天宝十二年（公元 753 年）11 月 15 日，他率弟子 40 余人第 6 次启程渡海，同年在日本萨摩秋妻屋浦（今九州南部鹿儿岛大字秋月浦）登岸，经太宰府、大阪等地，于次年入日本首都平城京（今日本奈良），天皇派专使迎接，受到日本朝野僧俗的盛大欢迎。

## *Monk Jianzhen's 6-time voyage eastward to Japan*

In the 21$^{st}$ year of Kaiyuan Age of the Tang Dynasty (733 A.D.), Japan sent their Japanese monks Rongrui and Puzhao along with Tang envoys to study in China, and at the same time invited Chinese eminent monks to teach in Japan. In the 1$^{st}$ year of Tianbao Age (742 A.D.), Jian Zhen accepted the invitation of Japanese monks. In the 2$^{nd}$ year of Tianbao Age (743 A.D.), Jianzhen together with his disciples Xiangyan, Daoxing and others began to cross the East. Within 10 years, they tried to cross the ocean for 5 times through all the difficulties but failed. After the failure of the fifth eastward voyage, the 62-year-old Jianzhen Master was blind. His eldest disciple, Xiangyan, died of illness and the Japanese monk who had invited him also died. However, he never gave up. In the 12$^{th}$ year of Tianbao Age of the Tang Dynasty (753 A.D.) on November 15, he led more than 40 disciples on their 6$^{th}$ journey across the sea. In the next year, he arrived at Japanese Capital Nara, where he was greeted by an envoy sent by the Japanese Emperor and warmly welcomed by the Japanese monks and society.

# 32

# 王怀隐《太平圣惠方》的针灸内容

Contents of acupuncture and moxibustion in WANG Huai-yin's *Taiping Shenghui Fang (Formulas from Benevolent Sages Compiled during the Taiping Era)*

王怀隐（约公元 925—997 年），宋州睢阳（今河南商丘）人。王怀隐最早为道士，擅长医术，后奉诏还俗，任命为尚药奉御，升至翰林医官使。

宋淳化三年（公元 992 年），王怀隐等奉诏编撰成《太平圣惠方》100 卷，虽然第 1~98 卷涉及针灸内容甚少，但第 99 卷则以论述针法为主，第 100 卷又是灸法专论，并附有经络腧穴图，对保存已佚文献及发展针灸医学都有较大贡献，是继《外台秘要》之后内容较好，有一定特色，又比较珍贵的针灸文献。

WANG Huai-yin (about 925–997 A.D.) was a man of Suiyang of Songzhou (currently, Shangqiu of Henan Province). In his early years, he was a Taoist priest and was good at medical skills. Later, he accepted the imperial edict to resume his secular life, and was appointed to be an aulic apothecary serving the emperor, and was promoted to be a "Hanlin Yiguan Shi" (medical official) in the imperial academy.

In the 3rd year of Chunhua Age of the Song Dynasty (992 A.D.), WANG Huai-yin and his colleagues accepted the imperial edict to write the book *Taiping Shenghui Fang* (《太平圣惠方》 *Formulas from Benevolent Sages Compiled during the Taiping Era*) with 100 volumes, of which Volume 1–98 contain fewer contents on acupuncture and moxibustion, but, Volume 99 mainly focuses on acupuncture techniques, and the Volume 100 is a treatise on moxibustion and has illustrations showing meridians and acupoints. These data are quite valuable and have certain characteristics following *Waitai Miyao*. They are the supplement of the lost literature in China and contribute a lot to the development of acupuncture-moxibustion medicine.

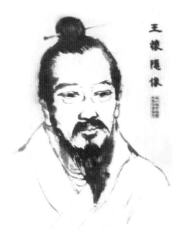

◇王怀隐画像

引自《中国历代名医图传》(陈雪楼主编,江苏科学技术出版社,1987年)

WANG Huai-yin's portrait
Cited from book *Zhongguo Lidai Mingyi Tuzhuan* (Editor-in-chief CHEN Xue-lou, published by Jiangsu Science and Technology Press in 1987)

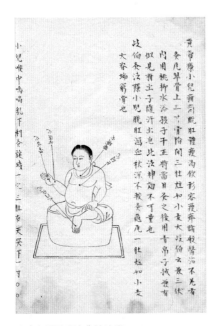

◇《太平圣惠方》针法卷

日本抄本

Volume Acupuncture Techniques in book *Taiping Shenghui Fang*
The Japanese transcript

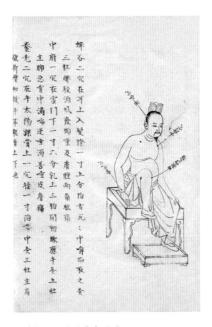

◇《太平圣惠方》灸法卷

日本抄本

Volume Moxibustion in book *Taiping Shenghui Fang*
The Japanese transcript

# 33

# 王惟一与《铜人腧穴针灸图经》

WANG Wei-yi and *Tongren Shuxue Zhenjiu Tujing (Illustrated Manual of Acupoints of the Bronze Figure)*

　　王惟一,又名王惟德,生于北宋太宗雍熙四年(公元987年),卒于北宋英宗治平四年(公元1067年),北宋著名针灸医家。

　　北宋天圣四年(公元1026年),王惟一撰成《铜人腧穴针灸图经》3卷。该书重新考订明堂腧穴,统一了腧穴的位置和所属经脉,增补了腧穴的主治病证。随后,宋政府将此书颁行全国作为教材,同时将之刻于石碑之上,以备观览。天圣五年(公元1027年),王惟一奉旨铸造了两具中国官方历史上最早的针灸铜人——宋天圣针灸铜人,供针灸教学使用。

WANG Wei-yi, also called WANG Wei-de, was born in the 4<sup>th</sup> year of Yongxi Age of the Emperor Taizong of the Northern Song Dynasty (987 A.D.), and died in the 4<sup>th</sup> year of Zhiping Age of Emperor Yingzong of the Northern Song Dynasty (1067 A.D.). He was a famous acupuncturist at that time.

In the 4<sup>th</sup> year of Tiansheng Age of the Northern Song Dynasty (1026 A.D.), WANG Wei-yi wrote the book *Tongren Shuxue Zhenjiu Tujing* (《铜人腧穴针灸图经》 *Illustrated Manual of Acupoints of the Bronze Figure*) with 3 volumes in which the Mingtang acupoints were re-verified and revised, their locations and the pertained meridians were unified. Moreover, clinical indications of the acupoint were supplemented. Afterwards, the Song Dynasty government issued an order to take this book as a national teaching material, and simultaneously, to carve it onto a stone tablet for people to view and read. In the 5<sup>th</sup>

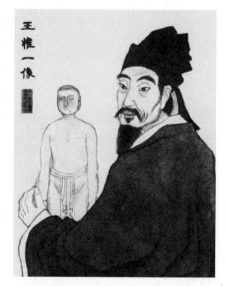

◇王惟一画像

引自《中国历代名医图传》(陈雪楼主编,江苏科学技术出版社,1987年)

WANG Wei-yi's portrait
Quoted from book *Zhongguo Lidai Mingyi Tuzhuan* (Editor-in-chief CHEN Xue-lou, published by Jiangsu Science and Technology Press in 1987)

year of Tiansheng Age (1027 A.D.), WANG Wei-yi accepted the imperial order to cast two bronze statues, Tiansheng Acupuncture Bronze Figures—the earliest bronze figures on acupuncture used for demonstration in teaching practice.

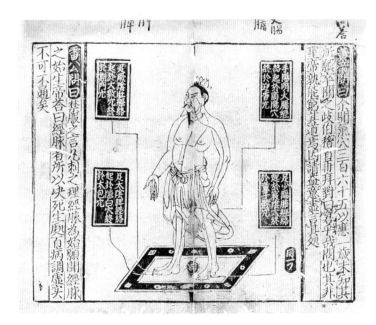

◇《铜人腧穴针灸图经》经脉图

元刊本,台湾中央图书馆藏

Meridian diagram from *Tongren Shuxue Zhenjiu Tujing*
Block-printed edition of the Yuan Dynasty, reserved by Taiwan Central Library

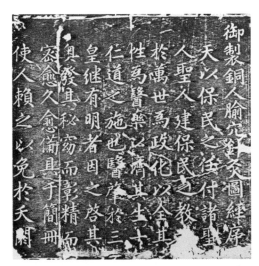

◇《铜人腧穴针灸图经》石刻拓片

明正统八年,日本宫内厅书陵部藏

Stone inscription rubbings of *Tongren Shuxue Zhenjiu Tujing*
Made in the 8th year of Zhengtong Age of the Ming Dynasty, preserved by the Library of Palace Inner Hall of Japan

# 34

# 宋天圣针灸铜人
## Tiansheng Acupuncture Bronze Figure of the Song Dynasty

　　宋天圣铜人是我国官方历史上最早的针灸铜人。北宋王惟一在完成《铜人腧穴针灸图经》后，奉旨根据该书于天圣五年（公元 1027 年）铸造成两具针灸铜人。铜人外刻经络腧穴，内置脏腑，以作针灸教学、医疗和考核之用。这种直观的教学模型是实物形象教学法的重大发明，是宋代医学教育的一大创举，对针灸学的发展有着深远影响。

　　明代正统八年（1443 年）时，宋天圣铜人身上的穴位已模糊难辨，明英宗下令严格依照宋天圣铜人复制一具新铜人，复制成功后的铜人被称为"明正统铜人"。然而就在明正统铜人铸成后，宋天圣铜人突然间没有了踪迹，关于它的去向之谜有多种猜测。

　　Tiansheng bronze figure of the Northern Song Dynasty is the earliest acupuncture figure in Chinese official history. Following completing book *Tongren Shuxue Zhenjiu Tujing*, WANG Wei-yi took the imperial decree to cast two bronze figures in the 5th year of Tiansheng Age (1027 A.D.). These bronze figures, engraved with meridians and acupoints at the body surface and with Zang-fu organs in the interior, were used for teaching, medical treatment and examination of acupuncture and moxibustion. This macroscopic teaching model is a great invention of entity image teaching method, a great pioneering work in medical education of the Song Dynasty, and has a far-reaching impact on the development of acupuncture and moxibustion teaching.

　　In the 8th year of Zhengtong Age of the Ming Dynasty (1443 A.D.), the acupoint locations on Tiansheng Acupuncture Bronze Figure were indistinguishable. So, Emperor Yingzong ordered to duplicate a new bronze figure in accordance with Tiansheng Acupuncture Bronze Figure which was called as "Ming Zhengtong Acupuncture Bronze Figure". Thereafter, the Tiansheng Acupuncture Bronze Figure disappeared unexpectedly, which arose a lot of speculations about its whereabouts.

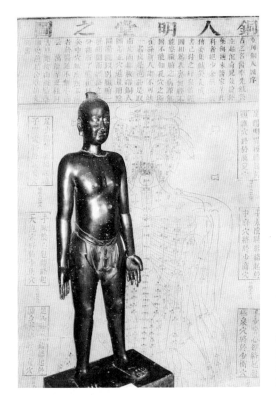

◇明正统仿宋针灸铜人

**俄罗斯圣·彼得堡国立艾尔米塔什博物馆藏**

Zhengtong Acupuncture Bronze Figure of the Ming Dynasty, a copied Song Dynasty's acupuncture bronze figure, preserved in St. Petersburg State Hermitage Museum of Russia

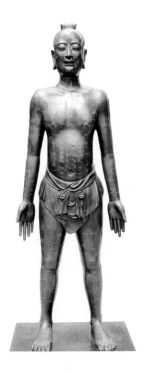

◇明正统仿宋针灸铜人（复制品）

**2002 年复制，中国中医科学院针灸研究所针灸博物馆藏**

Zhengtong Acupuncture Bronze Figure of the Ming Dynasty, a copied Song Dynasty's acupuncture bronze figure (replica) Duplicated in 2002, preserved in the Chinese Museum of Acupuncture and Moxibustion, Institute of Acupuncture and Moxibustion, CACMS

## 宋天圣铜人的下落之谜

　　宋天圣铜人铸成后，一具放置在医官院，一具放置在大相国寺。约一百年后，即北宋末年靖康之乱（公元1126年），首都汴京（今河南开封市）失陷于金人，当时在汴京的这两具铜人也都相继流落到民间。《齐东野语》记载，其中一具针灸铜人辗转流落至襄阳（今湖北襄阳一带），后来由赵南仲重新献回南宋政府。南宋政府保留了很短的时间，就于公元1233年因战败将针灸铜人转送给蒙古政府。《元史》记载，元中统年间（公元1260—1263年）蒙古政府请工匠阿尼哥修整过此铜人。此后不久，蒙古政府将铜人由汴京转移至京师天顺府（今北京）三皇庙，后又移入宫中。明正统八年，明英宗下令铸制了一具针灸铜人，即明正统铜人。正统铜人铸成后，天圣铜人下落不明，有的学者认为是在明代的某次战争中被毁灭的。

## The mystery of whereabouts of Tiansheng bronze figure of the Song Dynasty

After the founding of the Tiansheng bronze figures, one was placed in the medical officials' academy, another in Daxiangguo Temple. About a hundred years later, during the Jingkang Rebellion (1126 A.D.) in the late Northern Song Dynasty, the capital of Bianjing (now Kaifeng City, Henan Province) fell into the Jin nationality. At the same time, the two bronze figures in Bianjing went to the public successively. *Qidong Yeyu* (《齐东野语》*Civilian Saying of Eastern Qi State*) records that one of the acupuncture bronze figures wandered to Xiangyang (Xiangyang, Hubei Province currently), and later returned to the Southern Song government by ZHAO Nan-zhong. The government of the Southern Song Dynasty kept it only for a very short period of time, and in 1233 A.D., after the failure of war, the bronze figure was transferred to the Mongolian government. *Yuanshi* (《元史》*The History of the Yuan Dynasty*) recorded that the Mongolian government asked the craftsman Aniko to repair the bronze figure during Zhongtong Age of the Yuan Dynasty (1260–1263 A.D.). Shortly thereafter, the Mongolian government transferred the bronze figure from Bianjing to Sanhuang Imperial Temple of the capital Tianshunfu (now Beijing) and later to the palace. In the 8th year of Zhengtong Age of the Ming Dynasty, the emperor Yingzong ordered to duplicate a new bronze figure called Ming Zhengtong Acupuncture Bronze Figure. After Zhengtong bronze figure was made, whereabouts of Tiansheng bronze figure became a mystery. Some scholars have believed that it was destroyed in a war in the Ming Dynasty.

# 35

## 杨介与经络图
YANG Jie and the meridian diagram

　　杨介,字吉老,泗州(今江苏省盱眙县)人,约生于北宋熙宁元年(公元 1068 年),卒于南宋绍兴十年(公元 1140 年),著名医家。

　　北宋政和二年(公元 1112 年),杨介著成《存真图》一卷,后增加十二经脉之图、文,合为《存真环中图》一书,于公元 1113 年刊行。其中,"存真"即脏腑图,对人体脏腑作了详细的解剖描述;"环中"即十二经脉图,是宋代较为完整、典型的经脉图。《存真环中图》对后世解剖学和针灸学的发展影响深远。该书惜佚,但其内容通过日本医籍《万安方》《顿医抄》的转载而得以保存。

　　YANG Jie, courtesy name Jilao, a native of Sizhou (current Xuyi County of Jiangsu Province), a famous physician of the Song Dynasty, was born in the first year of Xining Age of the Northern Song Dynasty (1068 A.D.) and died in the 10th year of Shaoxing Age of the Southern Song Dynasty (1140 A.D.).

In the 2nd year of Zhenghe Age of the Northern Song Dynasty (1112 A.D.), YANG Jie completed the 1st volume of book *Cunzhen Tu* (《存真图》*Pictures of Reserving the True*); afterwards, he supplemented illustrations and legends of the twelve meridians and combined them together to compose a complete book *Cunzhen Huanzhong Tu* (《存真环中图》*Pictures of Circulatory Courses of Meridians and the Internal Organs*) which was printed and published in 1113 A.D. The word "Cunzhen" means the diagrams of the internal organs, giving a detailed description on the anatomical structure of the human viscera; while the word "Huanzhong" refers to the diagrams of circulatory courses of the 12 regular meridians, which are the relatively intact and typical diagrams of the twelve regular meridians of the Song Dynasty. The book *Cunzhen Huanzhong Tu* has a profound influence on the development of the ancient anatomy and acupuncture-moxibustion medicine of the later generations. Despite of being lost in China, its related contents are reserved via the transcripts of Japanese medical book *Wan-an Fang* (《万安方》*Formulary for Absolute Safety*) and *Dunyi Chao* (《顿医抄》*Essentials of Medicine*).

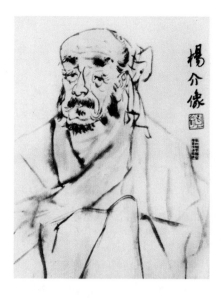

◇杨介画像
　引自《中国历代名医图传》（陈雪楼主编，江苏科学技术出版社，1987 年）

YANG Jie's portrait
Cited from book *Zhongguo Lidai Mingyi Tuzhuan* (Editor-in-chief CHEN Xue-lou, published by Jiangsu Science and Technology Press in 1987)

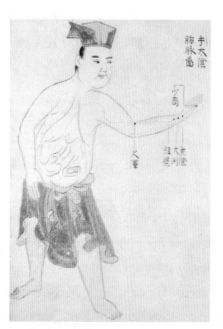
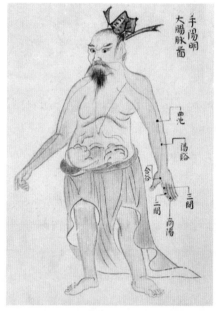

◇手太阴肺脉图和手阳明大肠脉图
　引自日本医籍《万安方》

Diagrams of the Lung Meridian of Hand-taiyin and the Large Intestine Meridian of Hand-yangming
Cited from Japanese medical book *Wan-an Fang*

# 36

## 《黄帝针经》北宋回归

## Return of *Huangdi Zhenjing* (*The Yellow Emperor's Classic on Acupuncture*) in the Northern Song Dynasty

　　宋金元时期,中国医书传至朝鲜日益增多,有些在中国已难看到或散佚的医书,在朝鲜得以完好保存。这些书大多由民间传去,或由朝鲜刻版印刷而保留下来。

　　宋元祐六年(公元 1091 年),宋哲宗令人抄录一批医药书目交与回国的高丽使者,计有《黄帝针经》《黄帝九墟经》《黄帝内经太素》《陈延之小品方》《甄权古今录验方》等。宋元祐七年(公元 1092 年),高丽宣宗帝派遣使者入宋,携带中国所缺而朝鲜尚存之善本医书回献宋王朝,其中尤以善本《黄帝针经》九卷得众瞩目。至此,这部在隋唐时已佚,至宋时已数百年不见的针灸典籍,又得以在中国流传。这是朝鲜对中国医学的重要贡献,也反映出两国在针灸医学方面的互相交流情况。

In the period of Song, Jin and Yuan Dynasties, more and more Chinese medical works were spread to the North Korea. Some medical books were rarely seen or lost in China, but are preserved perfectly in North Korea. Most of these books were spread there through the civilians or reserved by North Korean block-printing thereafter.

In the 6th year of Yuanyou Age of the Song Dynasty (1091 A.D.), Emperor Zhezong issued an order to transcribe a list of medical books to give a Korean envoy who was going to his home country. The booklist included *Huangdi Zhenjing* (《黄帝针经》*The Yellow Emperor's Classic on Acupuncture*), *Huangdi Jiuxu Jing* (《黄帝九墟经》*The Yellow Emperor's Inner Classic in Nine Parts*), *Huangdi Neijing Taisu* (《黄帝内经太素》*Grand Simplicity of 'The Yellow Emperor's Inner Classic*), *Chen Yan-zhi's Xiaopin Fang* (《陈延之小品方》*CHEN Yan-zhi's Prescriptions in Brief*), *Zhenquan Gujin Lu Yanfang* (《甄权古今录验方》*ZHEN Quan's Proven Priscriptions from the Past and Present*), etc. In the 7th year of Yuanyou Age of the Song Dynasty (1092 A.D.), the Korean emperor dispatched an envoy to carry medical books (which had been lost in China but reserved in Korea) to China and give them back to the Song Government. *Huangdi Zhenjing* with 9 volumes, one of the rare books, gained lots of attention from people at that time. So far, this ancient Chinese book on acupuncture and moxibustion that had been lost in the period of Sui and Tang Dynasties and had disappeared for several hundreds years till the Song Dynasty, was spread again in ancient China. This is an important contribution of North Korea to Chinese medicine. It also reflects the mutual interchange situations in acupuncture and moxibustion between the two countries.

十八

嘉祐四年，仁宗謂輔臣曰：「宋、齊、梁、陳、後魏、北齊書，世罕有善本，未行之學官，可委編校官精加校勘。」八月，命編校書籍孟恂、丁寶臣、趙彥若、錢藻、孫覺、曾鞏校宋、齊、梁、陳、後魏、北齊、後周七史。拘等言：「梁、陳等書缺，獨館閣所藏，恐不足以定著，願詔京師及州縣藏書之家，使悉上之。」仁宗皇帝爲下其事，至七年冬，稍稍始集，然後校正訛繆，遂爲完書，模本行之。

十九

嘉祐六年四月，以大理寺丞郭固編校祕閣所藏兵書。先是，三館祕閣置官編校書籍，而兵書與天文爲祕書，獨不預。大臣有言固曉知兵法，仍命就祕閣編校，抄成黃本一百七十二冊。固初以選換六宅副使，治平四年六月，以編書畢，遷內藏庫副使、路分都監。

二十

哲宗時，臣察言：「竊見高麗獻到書，內有黃帝鍼經九卷。撰素問序稱，漢書藝文志黃帝內經十八篇，與此書各九卷，乃合本數。此書久經兵火，亡失幾盡，偶存於東夷。今此來獻，篇帙具存，不可不宣布海內，使學者誦習。伏望朝廷詳酌，下尚書工部，雕刻印板，送國子監依例摹印施行。所貴濟

卷第三十一　兩朝書籍

三九七

宋朝事實類苑

集之功，溥及天下。」有旨，令祕書省選奏通曉醫書官三兩員校對，及令本省詳定訖，依所申施行。

二十一

舊制，每日校對書籍功冊葉背面二十一紙，三館都監於每月終，具逐員功課聞奏。自嘉祐中置編校，此制途廢。元祐六年，復著爲令。又案六典，考工之職二十七，十日讎校精審。明於刊定，爲校正之最，乞以月終所奏，降付考功。詔依紹聖三年四月尚書省勘會館職，每日校對書籍，已有條制立定功課，即不須逐旋聞奏。其考功自來別無行遣，顯屬繁冗。奉聖旨，元祐六年指揮更不施行。

二十二

淳化元年二月，詔自今游宴，宣召直館，其集賢祕閣校理並令預會。初李宗諤舉進士，獻文自鬻，相府試詩頌各一篇，遷祕書郎集賢校理之職。自興國後，罕有任者。會帝宴近臣於後苑，三館學士悉預，宗諤逸其事，故有是詔。翌日獻詩述其事，不得入。又請令京官乘馬入禁門，並爲故事。

祖宗時，每時序游幸，或雨雪休應，皆賜宴于崇文院。祥符、天禧之際，宸章叡藻，宣示臣下，自宰執至貼職，皆得賡載。仁宗善飛白書，每賜臣下，館閣預焉。上巳、重陽，館閣賜宴于瑞聖園。

三九八

◇《宋朝事实类苑》中记载"《黄帝针经》北宋回归"

上海古籍出版社，1981 年

"Return of *Huangdi Zhenjing* in the Northern Song Dynasty" recorded in the book *Songchao Shishi Leiyuan* (《宋朝事实类苑》*Interesting Historical Stories and Fantastic Poems of the Song Dynasty*) Published by Shanghai Ancient Book Publishing House, in 1981

##  《黄帝针经》回归故里

　　《宋朝事实类苑》卷31记述："哲宗时，臣僚言：窃见高丽献到书，内有《黄帝针经》九卷。据《素问》序称，《汉书·艺文志》'《黄帝内经》十八篇'。《素问》与此书各九卷，乃合本数。此书久经兵火，亡失几尽，偶存于东夷。今此来献，篇帙具存，不可不宣布海内，使学者诵习。"可见，高丽所献之中国已佚经典《黄帝针经》在当时已引起朝野之高度重视，这对中国医学的发展是一件非常重要的补缺。在隋唐时，或更早时期，《黄帝针经》传至朝鲜，得到完整保存，于宋代再由朝鲜传回故乡中国，宋政府又视之为宝，迅即颁布天下，才使得该书又在中国流传。

## Return of Huangdi Zhenjing to the homeland

　　The 31st volume of *Songchao Shishi Leiyuan* records: "At the age of Zhezong, the Song Dynasty, an official says: Having seen accidentally the presentation of the book by Korean, including 9 volumes of *Huangdi Zhenjing*. According to the preface of *Suwen*, in *Hanshu: Yiwen Zhi*, there should be totally 18 chapters of *Huangdi Neijing*, 9 volumes of *Suwen*, and 9 volumes of *Zhenjing* for each. The book was lost during the war in China but reserved in Korea. The presented one is well preserved and should be spread widely for scholars to learn." It means that *Huangdi Zhenjing* presented by Korean at that time aroused great attention of the court and the commonalty, which has been a very important complement to the development of Chinese medicine. In the Sui and Tang Dynasties, or even earlier period, the lost book *Huangdi Zhenjing* was spread to Korea, where it had been well preserved, and returned to China in the Song Dynasty. The Song government regarded the book as a treasure and immediately issued a decree for popularization of the book in China.

# 37

# 宋太医局针科考试

Acupuncture examination of Imperial Medical Bureau in the
Song Dynasty

宋代政府注重医学教育,为提高教育质量,太医局逐步建立了一套完善的考试制度,学生常于春季应试。崇宁年间(公元 1102—1106 年),针科考试分三场:第一场考三经大义五题(三经是《素问》《难经》《黄帝三部针灸甲乙经》);第二场考小经大义三道(小经指《巢氏病源》《龙木论》《千金翼方》)、运气大义二题;第三场考假令治病三题。

宋代针科考试的试题及其答案保存在《太医局诸科程文》中,分为 6 类,共 87 道题,其中针灸类考题有 10 道,为我们具体考查宋代医学教育提供了珍贵的第一手资料。《太医局诸科程文》共九卷,由宋代太医局何大任所编,原书已佚,现存《四库全书》本系清代乾隆年间从《永乐大典》中辑出。

The Song government paid paticular attention to the medical education. In order to improve the quality of medical education, the Song Imperial Medical Bureau set up a set of consummate examination system. The students usually took the exams in the spring. In the Age of Chongning (1102–1106 A.D.), the acupuncture exam contained 3 tests. The first test was made up of 5 questions of "Sanjing Dayi" , of which the Sanjing (3 classical works) referred to *Suwen*, *Nanjing*, *Huangdi Sanbu Zhenjiu Jiayi Jing*, and "Dayi" referred to pathogenesis about abnormal changes of the natural world and Zang-fu organs of the human body and their interrelation. The second test included 3 questions of "Xiaojing Dayi" , of which 3 questions of the "Xiaojing" referred to those from 3 books: *Chaoshi Bingyuan* (《巢氏病源》*Chao's Treatise on Etiology*), *Longmu Lun* (《龙木论》*Nagajuna's Secret Treatise on Ophthalmology*), *Qianjin Yifang*, and 2 questions of "Yunqi Dayi" which referred to the doctrine on the five elements' motion and six kinds of natural factors. The 3$^{rd}$ test included 3 questions of "Jialing Zhibing" (to diagnose and treat diseases only according to texts).

The exam questions and answers of acupuncture subject in the Song Dynasty including 6 categories and 87 questions were preserved in book *Taiyiju Zhuke Chengwen* (《太医局诸科程文》

*Fixed Composition Forms in Official Exams of Various Subjects of the Imperial Medical Bureau*).
Among them, 10 exam questions belong to acupuncture. This book, composed of 9 volumes and
compiled by HE Da-ren of the Imperial Medical Bureau, provides us with valuable firsthand
materials for investigating medical education of the Song Dynasty. Unfortunately, the original book
has been lost, while the extant copy in *Siku Quanshu* (《四库全书》*Imperial Complete Collection of
Four book classifications*) was extracted from book *Yongle Dadian* (《永乐大典》*The Yongle Great
Encyclopedia*) in Emperor Qianlong Age of the Qing Dynasty.

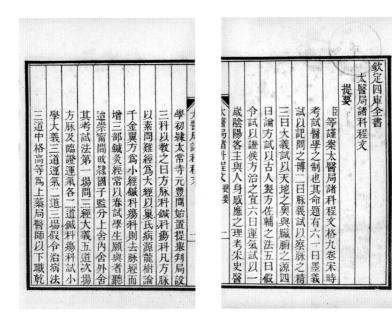

◇《太医局诸科程文》书影

《四库全书》本，中国中医科学院针灸研究所针灸博物馆藏

Photograph of *Taiyiju Zhuke Chengwen*

A copy from *Siku Quanshu*, collected by Chinese Museum of Acupuncture and Moxibustion,
Institute of Acupuncture and Moxibustion, CACMS

# 38

## 李唐"村医灸背图"
## LI Tang's "picture of a village-acupuncturist in performing moxibustion over the patient's back"

　　南宋著名画家李唐（约1049—1130年）画有一幅风俗题材的"村医灸背图"，生动地描绘了一位村医正在为背痈患者施行烧灼灸法，旁边的小童在准备膏药，以供灸后贴敷，又称"灸背图"。此图充分说明灸法在我国古代不仅用于内科、妇产科、小儿科疾病，而且广泛应用于外科痈疽发背疮疡等的治疗，亦是灸法在唐宋之际流传盛行的明证。

LI Tang (1049–1130 A.D.), a famous painter of the Southern Song Dynasty, painted a "picture of a village-acupuncturist in performing moxibustion over the patient's back" (a custom theme) on which a village-acupuncturist was performing scorching moxibustion over the back of a patient with carbuncle, and a child nearby was preparing some medical paste for local application after the treatment. It is also called as "Body Back-moxibustion Picture". This picture fully indicates that moxibustion is not only applied to treatment of problems of the internal medicine, the department of gynecology and obstetrics, pediatrics, etc., but also to surgical conditions such as pyocutaneous disease, carbuncle of the back, etc. It is also a piece of evidence for extensive application of moxibustion in the periods of Tang and Song dynasties.

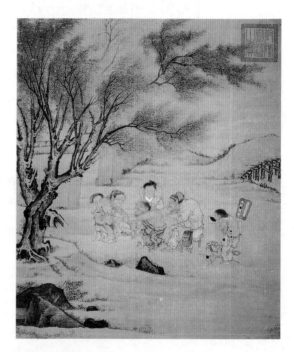

◇李唐"村医灸背图"
　中国台北故宫博物院藏

LI Tang's "picture of village-acupuncturist in performing moxibustion over the patient's back"
The original picture is preserved in Taipei National Palace Museum in Taiwan, China

# 39

# 窦材与《扁鹊心书》

DOU Cai and *Bianque Xinshu* ("*Bianque*"'s *Medical Experience*)

窦材,真定(今河北正定)人,约生于公元 1070 年,卒于公元 1146 年之后,南宋医家。

窦材出生于世医之家,早年曾任官职,后在衢州行医,晚年撰成《扁鹊心书》3 卷,该书为针、灸、药合一的著作。窦材临证擅用灸法,书中论述了百余种病证的灸法治疗,主张重灸、早灸,提倡大病宜灸、灸药同施等观点,指出应根据疾病的不同而选择灸量,强调顾护脾肾之阳,推崇保命要穴"关元"和"命关"。还创制"睡圣散"用于灸前麻醉,为多灸、重灸的患者减轻痛苦,这是他在运用灸法治病中最有特色的成就。

DOU Cai, a native of Zhending (current Zhengding City of Hebei Province), was born in about 1070 A.D. and died after 1146 A.D. He was a medical specialist of the Southern Song Dynasty.

DOU was born in a hereditary physician family of TCM. In his early years, DOU was once an official. Afterwards, he practiced medicine in Quzhou (current Quzhou of Zhejiang Province) district and wrote a book *Bianque Xinshu* (《扁鹊心书》"*Bianque*"'s *Medical Experience*, the "Bianque" here is in fact DOU's self-called name, not real Bianque) with 3 volumes in his late years. This book covers acupuncture, moxibustion (in particular) and materia medica. DOU Cai was well-known for his skillful techniques of moxibustion, and expounded treatment approaches of over one hundred of clinical problems with moxibustion in his book. He advocated that moxibustion should be applied in a larger dosage at the initial stage of illness, and in combination with medicinal herbs. Moreover, he also emphasized that the dosage of moxibustion should be given according to the concrete illness,

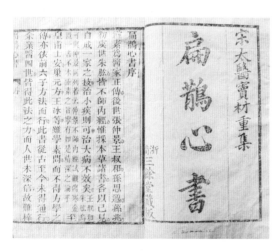

◇《扁鹊心书》书影

清刻本,中国中医科学院图书馆藏

Photograph of *Bianque Xinshu*
Block-printed edition of the Qing Dynasty, collected by the
Library of CACMS

and more attention should be paid to strengthening or protecting both spleen yang and kidney yang by needling Guanyuan (CV 4) and Mingguan. He invented a drug "Shuisheng San" (Powder for Inducing Sleep) for anesthesia before applying moxibustion so as to alleviate patients' sufferings during excessive and intensive moxibustion. This is his most distinctive achievement in practicing moxibustion.

 **三世扁鹊**

南宋名医窦材在其著作《扁鹊心书》中记载，一世扁鹊，乃黄帝时人，得岐黄血脉，曾授黄帝《太乙神明论》，著《五色脉诊》《三世病源》，后由淳于意、华佗所传承；二世扁鹊，乃战国时秦越人，撰《八十一难经》，每以扁鹊自比，谓医之正派，自号扁鹊；三世扁鹊，乃宋代窦材，自称得黄帝心法，革古今医人大弊，保天下苍生性命，常以扁鹊自任。

书中还载，窦材曾路过衢州野店，见一妇人遍身浮肿露地而坐，称土地爷说，有扁鹊过此，可求治病。窦材亦自称得扁鹊真传，有奇方，乃与妇人保命延寿丹内服，外灸左命关穴。妇人半月后痊愈，赞窦材乃"真扁鹊再生也"。

## Bianque in three different periods

*Bianque Xinshu*, compiled by DOU Cai, a famous physician of the Southern Song Dynasty, recorded that Bianque of the 1st period was born in the age of Huangdi, the Yellow Emperor. He ever studied and imparted *Taiyi Shenming Lun* (《太乙神明论》*Treatise on Taiyi Divinity*), compiled *Wuse Maizhen* (《五色脉诊》*Five Colors and Pulse Diagnosis*), *Sanshi Bingyuan* (《三世病源》*Origin of Diseases in Three Periods*), which were inherited later by physicians CHUNYU Yi and HUA Tuo; Bianque of the 2nd period refers to QIN Yue-ren, a physician in the the Warring States Period, who wrote the book *Bashiyi Nanjing*. He was honest and upright in medical practice and called himself Bianque; Bianque of the 3rd period refers to DOU Cai, a physician of the Song Dynasty, who called himself Bianque and believed that he learned the skills of TCM. He also advocated medical reform and put right the errors for protection of human life.

The book also recorded that DOU Cai once passed through Quzhou and saw a woman sitting in the open ground with edema all over the body, saying that she was told by the God of Earth if she could meet Bianque she would be cured. DOU Cai comforted the woman and told her that he had got a wonderful remedy handed down from Bianque. Then he prescribed the woman a formula of life-saving longevity pill and asked her to take it orally. In addition, he applied moxibustion at a point Mingguan on the left side externally. After half a month, the woman was cured and exclaimed that DOU Cai was a "reborn Bianque".

# 40

# 王执中与《针灸资生经》

## WANG Zhi-zhong and *Zhenjiu Zisheng Jing* (*Classic of Nourishing Life with Acupuncture and Moxibustion*)

王执中,字叔权,东嘉(今浙江省瑞安县)人,生卒年月不详,南宋乾道五年己丑(公元1169 年)中进士,曾任从政郎、将作丞,南宋著名针灸医家。

王执中参考《铜人腧穴针灸图经》《太平圣惠方》《千金要方》等书内容,约于公元1180—1195 年撰成《针灸资生经》7 卷,是一部文献价值、临床价值均较高的针灸书,对后世针灸学产生了较大的影响。书中详载腧穴的定位及取穴法,并将腧穴主治内容按病证类编,所以该书基本上是一部针灸腧穴专书。此外,书中阐述了作者对取穴、施灸、灸后护理、针灸禁忌以及针药关系等的独到见解。

WANG Zhi-zhong, courtesy name Shuquan, was a famous acupuncturist in the Southern Song Dynasty. He was a man of Dongjia (currently, Rui'an County of Zhejiang Province), but his birthday and death day remain unknown. In the 5th year of Qiandao Age of the Song Dynasty (1169 A.D.), he became a candidate in the highest imperial examination, and was once appointed as "Cong Zheng Lang" (从政郎), "Jiang Zuo Cheng" (将作丞, higher official).

Referring to the contents of books of *Tongren Shuxue Zhenjiu Tujing*, *Taiping Shenghui Fang* and *Qianjin Yaofang*, WANG wrote a book *Zhenjiu Zisheng Jing* (《针灸资生经》*Classic of Nourishing Life with Acupuncture and Moxibustion*) with seven volumes in about 1180–1195 A.D. This book introduced locations and selection methods of acupoints in detail, classified indications of acupoints according to the types of disorders, expounded the author's unique viewpoints on acupoints selection, moxibustion techniques, nursing after treatment with moxibustion, contraindications of both acupuncture and moxibustion, and the relationship between needling and medicine-herbal application, etc. Thus, it is actually an acupuncture monograph with high clinical value and high literature value, which produces a greater influence on the development of acupuncture and moxibustion in later generations.

◇《针灸资生经》书影

《四库全书》本，中国中医科学院图书馆藏

Photograph of *Zhenjiu Zisheng Jing*
A copy of *Siku Quanshu*, collected by the Library of CACMS

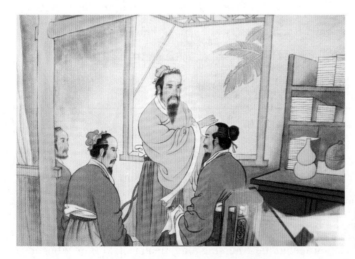

◇王执中灸上星穴治鼻衄

摄于湖南中医药大学针灸陈列馆

WANG Zhi-zhong was treating rhinorrhagia by
performing moxibustion at Shangxing (GV23)
Taken in the Museum of Acupuncture and
Moxibustion of Hunan University of TCM

# 41

# 宋代席氏家传针灸

## XI's family-handed down acupuncture-moxibustion in the Song Dynasty

席氏家传针灸,由宋到明,代代相传,历久不衰。其中,医名最显赫者,当属席氏针灸学派的创始人席弘。席弘,字弘远,号梓桑君,宋高宗南渡时席氏随着移居南方,安家于江西临川县,世代以针灸相传。

席弘以后,世代家传至十二世。此外,席弘十世孙席肖轩(字信卿)还把针灸术传给了外姓陈会。之后,陈会授徒24人,刘瑾是其中较为知名者。席氏门徒众多,遍及江西各地,形成了我国历史上较大的地区针灸派系——江西针灸学派。

XI's family's acupuncture-moxibustion techniques were handed down continuously for generations from the Song Dynasty to the Ming Dynasty, among whom, the most influential is XI Hong, the founder of XI's acupuncture-moxibustion school. XI Hong, courtesy name Hongyuan and alias Mr. Zisang, migrated to the southern China following Emperor Gaozong's crossing southwards in the Song Dynasty, and settled down in Linchuan County of Jiangxi Province.

In his family, acupuncture and moxibustion were handed down for 12 generations altogether. In addition, XI Xiao-xuan (courtesy name Xinqing), XI Hong's 10th generation's grandson, passed on his family's acupuncture skills to CHEN Hui (a man with surname other than XI's own). Afterwards, CHEN recruited 24 disciples, one of whom, LIU Jin was relatively well-known at that time. Many XI's disciples practiced acupuncture and moxibustion in every part of Jiangxi Province, forming Jiangxi acupuncture-moxibustion school, a larger regional acupuncture-moxibustion school in Chinese history.

| 席氏针灸世家传承关系 | |
| --- | --- |
| 席 弘 | 第一代 |
| 席灵阳 | 第二代 |
| 席玄虚 | 第三代 |
| 席洞玄 | 第四代 |
| 席松隐 | 第五代 |
| 席云谷 | 第六代 |
| 席素轩 | 第七代 |
| 席雪轩 | 第八代 |
| 席秋轩 | 第九代 |
| 席顺轩 ─ 席肖轩 | 第十代 |
| 席天章(子) 陈会(徒) | 第十一代 |
| 席伯珍 刘瑾 | 第十二代 |

◇席氏针灸世家传承关系
Inheriting relationship of XI's acupuncture-moxibustion family

## 席氏针灸传人陈会与《神应经》

陈会,字善同,别号宏纲先生,丰城横江里(今属江西)人,席氏针灸传人,明初针灸学家。陈会在长期的临床实践中,博采各家之长,撰成《广爱书》12卷,后经弟子刘瑾选录书中切合临床实用者重校成《神应经》1卷,刊于公元1425年。《神应经》一书取常用的119穴,采用歌诀与插图相配,方便阅读理解,并附以折量法、补泻口诀、取穴图说、诸病配穴以及针灸禁忌等。陈会临证针刺时,强调进出针手法,讲究催气候气方法,创用针刺"先泻后补"之法,形成了一套独特的针刺手法。

## CHEN Hui, successor of XI's acupuncture-moxibustion and Shenying Jing (《神应经》Classic of Acupuncture and Moxibustion with Obvious Therapeutic Tesults)

CHEN Hui, courtesy name Shantong, nickname Honggang, a native of Fengcheng (Jiangxi Province at present), was a successor of XI's acupuncture-moxibustion, an acupuncture expert in the early Ming Dynasty. In his long-term clinical practice, he had leaned experience of many physicians and scholars and compiled *Guang'ai Shu* (《广爱书》*Acupuncture-moxibustion Book of Diseases Treatment*) with 12 volumes. His disciple LIU Jin collected the practical part of the book, and reviewed it as *Shenying Jing* with only one volume, and had it published in 1425 A.D., which includes 119 commonly used points illustrated with charts and formulae in verse for better understanding matched with proportional measurement, methods of reinforcing and reducing, pictures for selecting points, point combination and acupuncture and moxibustion contraindications. In his clinical practice, CHEN Hui emphasized needling techniques of insertion and removal of the needles, as well as methods of promoting qi and waiting for the arrival of qi. He developed his unique needling technique of "reducing first and then reinforcing".

# 42

## 何若愚与子午流注针法
## HE Ruo-yu and Ziwu Liuzhu Zhenfa (midnight-noon ebb-flow needling)

从现存资料看,子午流注针法首见于金元时期何若愚的《流注指微针赋》,该文由阎明广作注,并收录于阎氏编撰的《子午流注针经》,是现存最早的子午流注专著。该书强调人体经脉气血的流注、开合随干支配合的不同日时而变化,系统论述了按时针刺的"子午流注法",提出了子午流注针法的两种取穴方法:纳甲法与养子时刻注穴法。后世医家王国瑞《扁鹊神应针灸玉龙经》中记载了"飞腾八法",徐凤《针灸大全》中记载了"灵龟八法"和"飞腾八法",高武《针灸聚英》中记载了纳子法的取穴方法,丰富和发展了子午流注针法。

By examing the existing documents, we can conclude that Ziwu Liuzhu Zhenfa (midnight-noon ebb-flow needling) in Chinese history was seen first in HE Ruo-yu's essay *Liuzhu Zhiwei Zhenfu* (《流注指微针赋》*Acupuncture Ode of the Subtleties of Flow*) during the Jin and Yuan Dynasties, for which YAN Ming-guang made annotations and included it in his book *Ziwu Liuzhu Zhenjing* (《子午流注针经》*Classic on Midnight-midday Acupuncture*), the existant earliest monograph about the doctrine of midnight-midday acupuncture. This monograph emphasizes regularly dynamic changes of the flowing, ebbing, open and close of qi and blood in human meridians along with different combinations of the 10 Heavenly Stems and the 12 Earthly Branches of the time (years, months, days and hours), systemically expounds the approaches of acupuncture treatment in the light of time-points of a day and puts forward two related methods of acupoint selection, i.e., Najia Fa (heavenly stem-preion of acupoint selection) and Yangxi Shike Zhuxue Fa (selection of acupoints according to the interpromotion of mother-son relationship, time, and flowing and ebbing of qi and blood). Thereafter, physicians of the later generations as WANG Guo-rui included Feiteng Bafa (eight methods for needling flying) in his book *Bianque Shenying Zhenjiu Yulong Jing* (《扁鹊神应针灸玉龙经》 *Bianque's Jade Dragon Classics of Acupuncture and Moxibustion*), XU Feng wrote down Linggui Bafa (eight methods of magic turtle) in his book *Zhenjiu Daquan*, and GAO Wu put forward Nazi Fa in his book *Zhenjiu Juying*. All of these greatly enrich and improve needling methods of Ziwu Liuzhu.

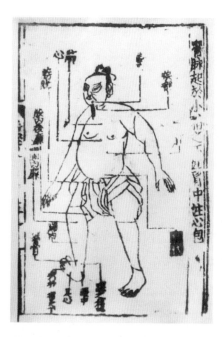

◇《子午流注针经》书影
《针灸四书》抄本转抄，中国中医科学院图书馆藏

Photograph of *Ziwu Liuzhu Zhenjing*
A transcribed copy of *Collection of 4 Books on Acupuncture and Moxibustion*,
collected by the Library of CACMS

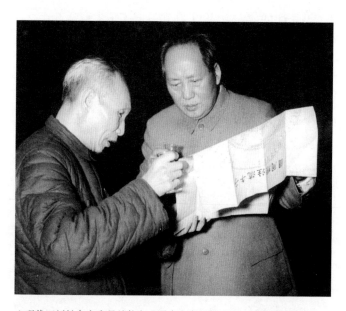

◇现代四川针灸名家吴棹仙向毛泽东主席呈献"子午流注环周图"

Mr.WU Zhao-xian, a well-known acupuncturist from Sichuan Province,
submitting a "Midnight-midday Circulating Diagram" to Chairman MAO Ze-
dong

# 43

# 闻人耆年与《备急灸法》

WENREN Qi-nian and *Beiji Jiufa (Moxibustion for Emergencies)*

闻人耆年,樵李(今浙江嘉兴西南)人,生活于 12—13 世纪之间,具体生卒年月不详,行医近四五十年,南宋针灸医家。

闻人耆年自幼习医,钻研典籍,涉猎诸家,于宋宝庆元年(公元 1226 年)撰成《备急灸法》。该书继承了葛洪和孙思邈用艾灸治疗急症的学术思想,结合自己的经验,论述了 22 种救急灸法,提出了一些常见危重病实用的抢救方法。他主张急症的治疗应早诊断、早施灸,艾灸量宜足,艾灸时取穴少,重在艾灸部位。书中还绘有 11 幅图谱,将病症所取的穴位(部位)标明在图上,依图取穴,方便实用。

WENREN Qi-nian, a native of Xieli (currently, the south-western part of Jiaxing of Zhejiang Province), was an acupuncturist of the Southern Song Dynasty. He lived in the 12th and 13th centuries but his birthday and death day remain unknown up to now. He practiced medicine for about 40–50 years.

WENREN started to learn medicine when he was a child, and intensively studied ancient books of various schools. He wrote *Beiji Jiufa* (《备急灸法》*Moxibustion for Emergencies*) in the 1st year of Baoqing Age of the Song Dynasty (1226 A.D.). This book inherits GE Hong's and SUN Si-miao's academic thoughts about treating emergencies with moxibustion and contains WENREN's own clinical experience. It expounds 22 types of moxibustion approaches for emergencies and summarizes some practical rescuing methods for some common and serious conditions. WENREN advocated that in the treatment of emergencies, earlier diagnosis, earlier moxibustion application, enough moxibustion dosage, fewer and suitable acupoints should be noted. This book has 11 illustrations with acupoint locations and related problems, being convenient and practicable in clinical practice.

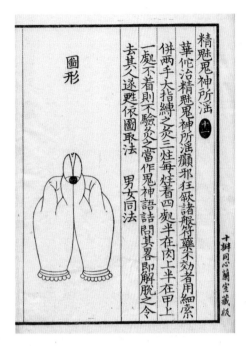

◇《备急灸法》书影
　影宋本，中国中医科学院图书馆藏

Photograph of *Beiji Jiufa*
Block-printed version of the Song Dynasty, collected by the Library of CACMS

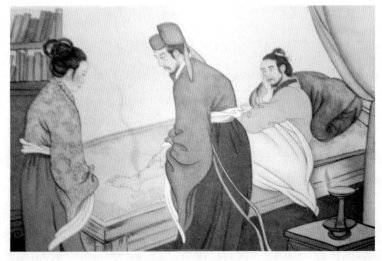

◇闻人耆年灸治风火牙痛
　摄于湖南中医药大学针灸陈列馆

WENREN Qi-nian treating acute toothache for a patient
Taken in the Museum of Acupuncture and Moxibustion of Hunan University of TCM

# 44

## 窦汉卿与窦氏针灸文集
## DOU Han-qing and his acupuncture books

　　窦汉卿,初名杰,字汉卿,后名默,字子声,广平肥乡（今河北肥乡县）人,生于金代明昌七年（公元 1196 年）,卒于元代至元十七年（公元 1280 年）,追授太师,谥文正,后人习称"窦太师""窦文正公",金元时期针灸名家。

　　窦氏在《内经》《难经》《铜人腧穴针灸图经》和《子午流注针经》等基础上,结合师传经验及其临床实践,撰成《标幽赋》《流注通玄指要赋》等,经窦桂芳辑校整理成《针经指南》（1312 年刊行）,体现了窦氏推崇毫针刺法、倡用"交经八穴"、阐发针刺补泻等的学术思想,对后世针灸学的发展起到了积极的推动作用。与窦太师相关的针灸文集还有《窦太师针经》《盘石金直刺秘传》等书。

DOU Han-qing, also named DOU Jie, courtesy name Hanqing in his early years, and DOU Mo, courtesy name Zisheng in his later years, a native of Feixiang of Guangping (current Feixiang County of Hebei Province). He was born in the 7th year of Emperor Mingchang Age of the Jin Dynasty (1196 A.D.), and passed away in the 17th year of Zhiyuan Age of the Yuan Dynasty (1280 A.D.). He was conferred with the imperial master after death by the emperor, with the temple title as "Wen Zheng". Thus, people often called him as "imperial master DOU" or "tutor Wenzheng DOU". He was a famous acupuncturist in the period of Jin and Yuan Dynasties.

　　Combining contents of *Huangdi Neijing*, *Nanjing*, *Tongren Shuxue Zhenjiu Tujing* and *Ziwu Liuzhu Zhenjing*, his tutor's experience and his own clinical practice, Master DOU wrote book *Biaoyou Fu* (《标幽赋》*Lyrics of Recondite*

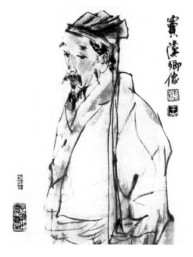

◇窦汉卿画像

引自《中国历代名医图传》（陈雪楼主编,江苏科学技术出版社,1987 年）

DOU Han-qing's portrait
Cited from book *Zhongguo Lidai Mingyi Tuzhuan* (Editor-in-chief CHEN Xue-lou, published by Jiangsu Science and Technology Press in 1987)

*Principles*) and *Liuzhu Tongxuan Zhiyao Fu* (《流注通玄指要赋》*Ode of the Essentials for Penetrating Mysteries*), etc. which were then composed into a book *Zhenjing Zhinan* (《针经指南》*A Guide to the Classic of Acupuncture*) after revision and rearrangement by DOU Gui-fang (published in 1312 A.D.). This revised book fully embodies Master DOU's needling techniques of filiform needles, application of the eight influential acupoints, and academic thoughts about reinforcing and reducing needling techniques of acupuncture, promoting the development of acupuncture and moxibustion of the later generations. Moreover, there are also some other books as *Doutaishi Zhenjing* (《窦太师针经》*Master Dou's Acupunture Classics*), *Panshijin Zhici Michuan* (《盘石金直刺秘传》 *Panshijin Esoteric Techniques on Perpendicular Insertion of Needle*), etc. related to imperial master DOU.

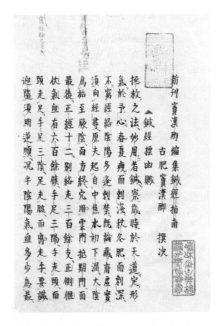

◇《针经指南》书影

日本抄本，中国中医科学院图书馆藏

Photograph of *Zhenjing Zhinan*
The Japanese transcript, collected by the Library of CACMS

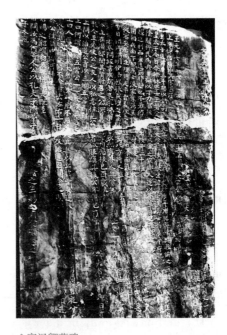

◇窦汉卿墓碑

位于河北省邯郸市

DOU Han-qing' gravestone
Located in Handan City of Hebei Province

**窦氏针法传人王国瑞**

　　王国瑞,元朝婺源(今浙江省兰溪)人,约生活在 13 世纪末至 14 世纪中叶,元代著名针灸学家,窦汉卿的再传弟子。撰有《扁鹊神应针灸玉龙经》一卷,刊行于元文宗天历二年(公元 1329 年),其主体部分"玉龙歌"及其注文是一篇总结临床经验且易传诵的歌赋。其学术思想主要源自金元时期何若愚、窦汉卿一派,在继承窦氏针法的基础上,重视气血流注盛衰与针灸时间的关系,发展了子午流注针法,创立了"飞腾八法"。针法方面,强调针灸并用、补泻兼施,是重视手法派的前驱。

## WANG Guo-rui, successor of DOU's acupuncture techniques

　　WANG Guo-rui, a native of Wuyuan (current Lanxi City, Zhejiang Province), in the Yuan Dynasty, lived from the end of the 13th century to the middle of the 14th century. He was a famous acupuncturist and the second-generation disciple of DOU Han-qing. He compiled one volume of *Bianque Shenying Zhenjiu Yulong Jing* and had it published in the 2nd year of Tianli Age of the Yuan Dynasty (1329 A.D.). The main part *Yulong Ge* (*Song of Jade Dragon*) with annotations was an ode easy to be recited that had summarized clinical experience. His academic thoughts mainly originated from HE Ruo-yu and DOU Han-qing in the Jin and Yuan Dynasties. On the basis of inheriting DOU's acupuncture techniques, he attached importance to the relationship between the excess and deficiency of qi and blood flow and chronological acupuncture, developed the needling therapy of midnight-noon ebb-flow and "eight methods of intelligent turtle" and emphasized the combination of acupuncture and moxibustion, as well as reinforcing-reducing methods. He was a pioneer in emphasizing the needling techniques.

# 45

# 滑寿与《十四经发挥》

HUA Shou and *Shisi Jing Fahui* (*An Elucidation of the Fourteen Meridians*)

滑寿,字伯仁,晚号撄宁生,祖籍河南襄城,约生于元大德八年(公元1304年),卒于明洪武十九年(公元1386年),元末明初著名医家。

滑寿幼年习儒书于韩说先生,后弃科举而钻研医术,撰有《十四经发挥》3卷,是滑寿在元代针灸学家忽泰必烈《金兰循经取穴图解》一书的基础上补注、改编而成,刊行于公元1341年。该书考订腧穴,详加训释,重视任督二脉,提出任督二脉与十二经并称十四经学说。书中将腧穴的归经、排列次序与经络循行的方向、路线紧密联系,对人体十四经脉的循行进行了较为详细的注释,确定了以十四经脉为统领的腧穴分类排列形式,是一本研究经脉的专书,对后世针灸腧穴学产生了深远影响。

HUA Shou, courtesy name Boren, and alias Ying ningsheng during his later years, was born in Xiangcheng of Henan Province in about the 8<sup>th</sup> year of Dade Age of the Yuan Dynasty (1304 A.D.) and died in the 19<sup>th</sup> year of Hongwu Age of the Ming Dynasty (1386 A.D.). He was a famous physician between the late period of Yuan Dynasty and the early stage of Ming Dynasty.

During his young age, HUA Shou learned Confucianism from tutor HAN Shuo. Later, he gave up imperial examinations and began to devote himself to medical skills. After supplementing, revising and recomposing *Jinlan Xunjing Quxue Tujie* (《金兰循经取穴图解》*Gold Orchid Book with Illustrations for Selecting Points along Meridians*) written by Hutai Bi-lie, a senior acupuncturist of the Yuan Dynasty, he wrote a book *Shisi Jing Fahui* (《十四经发挥》*An Elucidation of the Fourteen Meridians*) with 3 volumes and published it in 1341 A.D. In this book, he systematically investigated and revised the extant acupoints at that time, made detailed explanations about them, paid a particular attention to the Conception and Governor vessels, and put forward a doctrine of 14 meridians (12 regular meridians and Conception and Governor vessels). Additionally, he especially made the meridian distribution, running directions and routes and the acupoints' meridian-tropism and arrangement sequence link closely, gave a detailed annotation on the running routes of the 14 meridians in the human body, and established a classification and arrangement style of acupoints by taking the 14 meridians as the leading lines. This book is a monograph on meridians and brings about far-reaching influence on the acupoint learnings of the later generations.

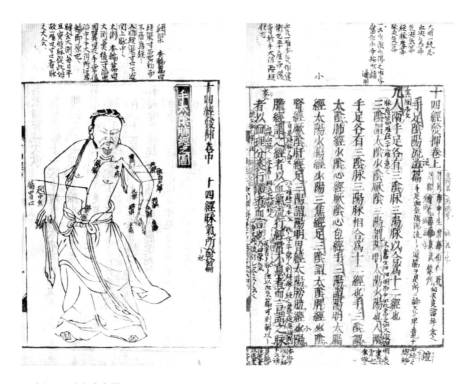

◇《十四经发挥》书影

   日本刊本，协和医科大学图书馆藏

Photograph of *Shisi Jing Fahui*

Japanese block-printed version, collected by the Library of Peking Union Medical University

# 46

## 日本针灸铜人和铜人图
Japanese acupuncture bronze figure and its picture

明朝初期日本来华的留学生竹田昌庆,于明洪武十一年(公元 1378 年),在中国购置一具小型针灸铜人带回日本,日本医家视之如珍宝,对推动日本针灸学发展影响甚大。公元 1657 年(日本明历三年),日本遭受江户地区的大火,这一小铜人被毁灭。至此,传日针灸铜人在日本保存了长达 279 年之久。现日本东京国立博物馆中珍藏一具针灸铜人,视为国宝,有学者认为是中国北宋天圣针灸铜人流落到朝鲜后被日本掠去,亦有学者认为系日本幕府医学馆针灸医官奉幕府之命于 1809—1819 年间铸。

据 1936 年第 11 期《针灸杂志》载,日本帝室博物馆(现名东京国立博物馆)还藏有铜人腧穴像和日本宽永年制铜人像。1934 年秋,承澹盦先生赴日本考察期间,花巨资从日本购得铜人腧穴像照片 4 幅。

In the 11<sup>th</sup> year of Hongwu Age (preliminary stage) of the Ming Dynasty (1378 A.D.), a Japanese student Takeda Changkei who was studying in China, purchased a mini-acupuncture bronze figure and brought it back to Japan. This bronze figure drew great attention in the Japanese medical circle, and has a bigger influence on the development of acupuncture medicine in Japan. In 1657 A.D. (the 3<sup>rd</sup> year of Japanese Mingli), this acupuncture bronze figure was damaged by a big fire in Edo area (current Tokyo), when it had been preserved for 279 years in Japan. Nowadays, another acupuncture bronze figure preserved in Tokyo National Museum is considered a Japanese national treasure. Some scholars believed that this extant acupuncture figure was the lost Chinese Tiansheng Acupuncture Bronze Figure built in the Northern Song Dynasty which was scattered to North Korea and then swept away by Japanese. Some other scholars believed that it was casted under the requirement of acupuncture officials from the Medical Institute of Japanese Medical Shogunate during 1809–1819.

According to the 11<sup>th</sup> issue of *Journal of Acupuncture and Moxibustion* in 1936, Japanese Imperial Museum (currently, Tokyo National Museum) also preserved a picture of acupoint bronze figure and a picture of bronze figure made in the Kuanyong Age of Japan. In the autumn of 1934 and during his visit in Japan, Mr. CHENG Dan-an paid a big sum of money to buy 4 pictures of the acupoint bronze figure.

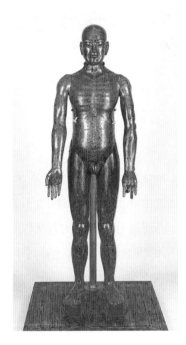

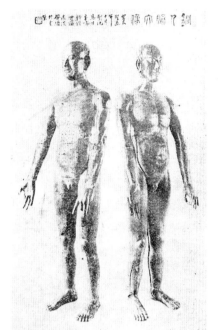

◇日本针灸铜人
　　日本东京国立博物馆藏

Japanese acupuncture bronze figure
Preserved in Tokyo National Museum of Japan

◇从日本所购铜人腧穴像（四幅之一）
　　引自 1936 年第 11 期《针灸杂志》

Acupoint bronze figure picture bought from Japan (one of the 4 pictures)
Cited from *Journal of Acupuncture and Moxibustion* (the 11th issue of 1936)

# 47

# 徐凤与《针灸大全》

XU Feng and *Zhenjiu Daquan* (*A Complete Work of Acupuncture and Moxibustion*)

徐凤,字廷瑞,号泉石,江右弋阳(今江西省弋阳县石塘)人,明代著名针灸医家。

徐凤学承金元时期的针灸名家窦汉卿派,结合自己数十年的临床经验,约于公元1439年撰成《针灸大全》6卷。该书汇集了明中期之前诸家,特别是金元针灸大师窦汉卿的针灸名篇,收有大量针灸歌赋,便于记诵。该书卷三《金针赋》即以歌赋形式详述补泻手法,重视针刺手法和按时取穴法,补充完善了子午流注针法,对后世针刺手法发展产生了深远影响,对明代针灸学的昌盛起到了推动作用。

XU Feng, courtesy name Tingrui and alias Quanshi, a native of Yiyang of Jiangyou (current Shitang of Yiyang County of Jiangxi Province), was a famous acupuncturist in the Ming Dynasty.

Combining DOU Han-qing school's thoughts of the Jin and Yuan Dynasties and his own clinical experience accumulated during the past several decades, XU Feng wrote 6 volumes of *Zhenjiu Daquan* (《针灸大全》*A Complete Work of Acupuncture and Moxibustion*) in 1439 A.D. His book collected abundant well-known writings of various academic schools before the mid-period of the Ming Dynasty, particularly those of Master DOU Han-qing. It also contained many rhymed proses of acupuncture and moxibustion for the convenience of easy-learning by heart. The ode, *Jinzhen Fu* (《金针赋》*Ode to Gold Needle*) of the 3rd volume of *Zhenjiu Daquan*, describes the reinforcing and reducing manipulations of acupuncture in detail, lays stress on needling techniques and time-determined acupoint selection, and supplements midnight-midday acupuncture techniques, playing an important influence on the development of acupuncture manipulations and the acupuncture-moxibustion medicine in the Ming Dynasty and the later generations.

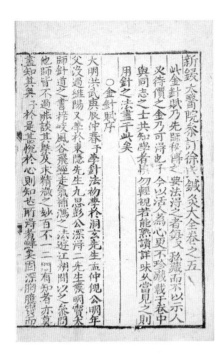

◇徐氏《针灸大全》书影

明末金陵三多斋刊本,中国中医科学院图
书馆藏

Photograph of XU's *Zhenjiu Daquan*
A block-printed edition of Sanduozhai of Jinling
(current Nanjing) in the late stage of Ming
Dynasty, collected by the Library of CACMS

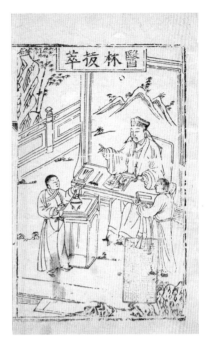

◇徐凤著书图

引自徐氏《针灸大全》

A picture of XU Feng in writing works
Taken from XU's *Zhenjiu Daquan*

# 48

# 明代针灸名医凌云
## LING Yun, a famous acupuncturist of the Ming Dynasty

凌云,字汉章,号卧岩,归安(今浙江省湖州)人,约生活于 15 世纪下半叶至 16 世纪上半叶,明代著名医家。

凌氏针法以针术精湛而著称于世,世代相传,虽未曾出版著作,但有写本传抄存世,存有《集英撮要针砭全书》《凌门传授铜人指穴》等,其中内容曾被《针灸聚英》等书引载。从现存写本中可知凌氏用穴和针法受金元针灸大师窦汉卿的影响较大,但在其基础上有所补充发挥,创立了独特的凌氏针法,可补窦氏理论之不足,是明代以来刺法运用的发展。

LING Yun, courtesy names Hanzhang, assumed name Woyan, a native of Gui'an (Huzhou of Zhejiang Province at present), lived in the later half of the 15th century and the former half of the 16th century. He was a famous physician of the Ming Dynasty.

LING's acupuncture techniques were well-known for his exquisite skills, and were handed down generations after generations. In spite of the fact of publishing no books, LING had some manuscript copies survived and handed down, such as *Jiying Cuoyao Zhenbian Quanshu* (《集英撮要针砭全书》 *A Complete Collection of Essential Gems on Needle-stone*), *Lingmen Chuanshou Tongren Zhixue* (《凌门传授铜人指穴》 *The Imparted Ling's School's Bronze Figure Showing Acupiont Locations*), etc. Some of their contents were cited by book *Zhenjiu Juying*, etc. We can know from the manuscripts that LING was influenced greatly by Master DOU Han-qing in acupoint selection and needling techniques. Moreover, he also created the unique LING's own needling techniques, making up for some weaknesses of DOU's theory and showing a progress of needling technique application since the Ming Dynasty.

治準繩為醫家所宗行履詳父樵傳
凌雲字漢章歸安人為諸生秉去北遊泰山古廟前遇
病人氣垂絕雲嗟歎久之一道人忽日汝欲生之乎日
然道人鍼其左股立蘇曰此人毒氣内侵非死也毒散
自生耳因授雲鍼術治疾無不效五日
眾投以補劑益甚雲曰此寒濕積也穴在頂鍼之必暈
絕逾時始蘇命四人分牽其髮使勿傾側乃鍼果暈絕
家人皆哭雲言笑自如頃之氣漸蘇復加補始出鍼嘔
積痰斗許病即除有男子病後舌吐雲兄亦知醫謂雲
不立效有本草集要名醫雜著行於世肯堂所著證

◇《明史·凌云传》书影

Photograph of book *Mingshi*: *Lingyun Zhuan* (*The History of the Ming Dynasty*: *The Biography of LING Yun*)

 ## 凌氏拜师学针术

凌云年轻时北游泰山古庙，遇到一个气息垂绝的病人，凌云很想救治，却束手无策，感慨良久。忽然来了一道人，问凌云，"你想让他活下来吗？"凌云说："当然。"于是，道人在病人的左侧大腿上针刺，病人立刻就苏醒过来了。道人给凌云讲解说，这个病人是因毒气内侵机体而致气息危绝，不是真的死了。针刺后，病人体内毒气散尽，就活过来了。凌云觉得道人针术高超，遂拜道人为师，潜心学习钻研针法，之后行医乡间，以针术闻名，治病几乎没有不见效的。

## *LING's story of learning acupuncture*

When LING Yun was young, he traveled north to the ancient temple of Mount Taishan. He met a patient who was in a critical condition of dying with feeble breath. LING Yun wanted to treat him but could do nothing. He sighed and felt helpless. Suddenly a Taoist priest came up and asked LING Yun, "Do you want him to live?" LING Yun said, "of course". So the priest punctured a point on the left thigh of the patient with a needle, and the patient came back to consciousness immediately. The priest explained to LIING Yun that the feeble breathing of the patient was due to invasion of the body by toxic pathogenic qi, which was not a real death. After the acupuncture treatment, the interior toxic pathogenic qi was dispersed and the patient came alive. LING Yun saw that the Taoist priest was experienced in acupuncture so he was apprenticed to him and devoted himself to learning and studying acupuncture. Being a famous acupuncturist, he practised medicine in the countryside later and seldom failed to treat the patients.

# 49

## 汪机与《针灸问对》
### WANG Ji and *Zhenjiu Wendui* (*Catechism on Acupuncture and Moxibustion*)

汪机（1463—1539 年），字省之，号石山居士，安徽祁门人，明代著名针灸学家。

汪机擅长针灸，一生著述很多，针灸著作有《针灸问对》3 卷。该书以《黄帝内经》《难经》《针灸甲乙经》等学术思想为依据，针对针灸学术领域存在的一些基本而又疑难的问题，设为 80 多条问答，所答者有据有理且有发挥，对有争议的问题，多能直言不讳，说出自己的看法，对误针、误灸的危害性，多能正言疾呼，对学者很有启发。

WANG Ji (1463–1539), courtesy name Shengzhi, assumed name Shishan Jushi (kulapati of Shishan Mountain), a native of Qimen of Anhui Province, was a famous acupuncturist of the Ming Dynasty.

WANG was versed in acupuncture and moxibustion skills and wrote a lot of writings in his whole life, including *Zhenjiu Wendui* (《针灸问对》*Catechism on Acupuncture and Moxibustion*) with 3 volumes. This book takes the academic thoughts of book *Huangdi Neijing*, *Nanjing* and *Zhenjiu Jiayi Jing* as the theoretical foundation, and sets up more than 80 problematic questions and answers in the field of acupuncture and moxibustion learnings. The answers are reasonable and have many new viewpoints. In regard to some debating questions, WANG often outspoke to utter his own viewpoints directly, and strongly warned the dangers of wrong needling and unreasonable moxibustion, which enlightens the related scholars a lot.

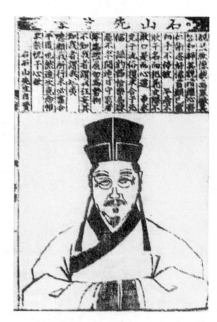

◇汪机画像
　引自《针灸问对》

WANG Ji's portrait
Cited from *Zhenjiu Wendui*

新安祁門朴墅汪機省之編輯
問邑門生石墅陳桷惟宜較正

针灸問對卷之上

或曰內經治病湯液醪醴為世少所載服餌之法統一
二而炎者四五其他則明針法無慮十八九厥後方藥
之說肆行而針炙之法僅而復存者何也
曰內經上古書也上古之人其知道乎勞不至倦逸不至
沈食不肥鮮以戕其內衣不蘊熱以傷其外起居有常寒
暑知避恬憺無為精神內守病雖有微風塵邪莫刈
能深入不過祭而已以針行滯散鬱刈
病隨已何待於湯液醪醴耶當今之世道德已衰以酒為
漿以妄為常縱欲以竭其精多慮以散其真不知持滿不

◇《针灸问对》书影
　明刊本，中国中医科学院图书馆藏

Photograph of *Zhenjiu Wendui*
Block-printed edition of the Ming Dynasty, collected by the
Library of CACMS

# 50

# 高武与《针灸节要聚英》
GAO Wu and *Zhenjiu Jieyao Juying* (*Extracted Collection of Gems in Acupuncture and Moxibustion*)

高武,号梅孤,四明(今浙江省宁波市鄞州区)人,约生活于 16 世纪,具体生卒年月不详,明代著名针灸学家。

高武早年善于骑射,应考武举失利,遂致力于医学,钻研针灸,于公元 1529—1537 年,先后撰成《针灸聚英》4 卷和《针灸节要》3 卷,作为《针灸节要聚英》一书的两个部分。《针灸节要》系节录《内经》《难经本义》有关针灸论述类编而成,《针灸聚英》撷取了历代医著中的针灸精华以及对针灸学的独特见解,是继汉代医家编《明堂经》首次全面总结腧穴主治症之后,又一次大规模的针灸腧穴文献辑录整理,对针灸学起着承先启后的作用,是一本学术价值较高的针灸专著,为后世针灸家所推崇。

他还亲自铸造针灸铜人 3 座,一男、一女、一幼,私铸铜人,在我国针灸史上较为少见。

GAO Wu, alias Meigu, a man of Siming (current Yin District of Ningbo City of Zhejiang Province), lived in about the 16th century, but his birthday and death day remain unknown. He was a famous acupuncturist of the Ming Dynasty.

GAO Wu was good at riding and archery in his early years, but failed in the provincial examinations of the military officer. He then devoted himself to medicine, particularly to the acupuncture and moxibustion learnings. From 1529 A.D. to 1537 A.D., he successively wrote 2 books *Zhenjiu Jieyao* (《针灸节要》*Extracted Gems in Acupuncture and Moxibustion*) with 3 volumes and *Zhenjiu Juying* (《针灸聚英》*A Collection of Gems in Acupuncture and Moxibustion*) with 4 volumes which are the two component parts of *Zhenjiu Jieyao Juying* (《针灸节要聚英》*A Collection of Extracts and Gems in Acupuncture and Moxibustion*). The *Zhenjiu Jieyao* was compiled from the excerpt of discourses in *Huangdi Neijing* and *Nanjin Benyi* (《难经本义》*The Genuine Meaning of the Classic on Difficult Problems*), and the latter *Zhenjiu Juying* absorbed the essences of acupuncture-moxibustion learnings and unique views from medical books of the past generations, which is once again a large-scaled literature compiling about acupuncture and moxibustion and acupoints after the first comprehensive summary of acupoint indications in *Huangdi Mingtang Jing* written by medical physicians of the Han Dynasty. It is thus a monograph on acupuncture and moxibustion with high academic value, serving as a link between the past and the future which is highly praised by the medical specialists of the later generations.

He personally casted 3 acupuncture bronze figures (one male, one female and one child), which has been seldomly seen in Chinese medical history.

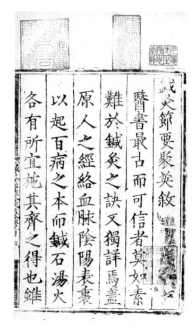

◇《针灸节要聚英》书影

　明刻本,中国中医科学院图书馆藏

Photograph of *Zhenjiu Jieyao Juying*
Block-printed edition of the Ming Dynasty,
collected by the Library of CACMS

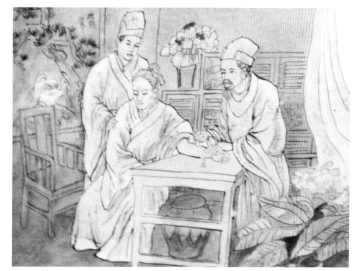

◇高武临证施灸

　摄于湖南中医药大学针灸陈列馆

GAO Wu performing moxibustion
Taken in the Museum of Acupuncture and Moxibustion of Hunan University of TCM

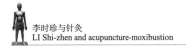
# 51

## 李时珍与针灸
LI Shi-zhen and acupuncture-moxibustion

李时珍,字东璧,号濒湖,蕲州(今湖北省蕲春县)人,生于明正德十三年(公元1518年),卒于明万历二十一年(公元1593年),明代杰出医药学家。

李时珍精通本草,一生著述丰厚,除撰有著名的《本草纲目》外,对经脉亦有研究,于公元1572年撰成《奇经八脉考》1卷。该书荟萃诸家之说,内容简要,篇目井然,不仅对奇经八脉分布路线进行了系统的整理,还阐述了其功能作用及基本病候,确立了奇经病证辨证论治的初步规范。该书是研究奇经八脉的珍贵文献资料,也是对经络理论的一大贡献。

LI Shi-zhen, courtesy name Dongbi, and alias Binhu, a native of Qizhou (current Qichun County of Hubei Province), was born in the 13th year of Zhengde regime (1518 A.D.) of the Ming Dynasty and passed away in the 21st year of Wanli regime of that dynasty (1593 A.D.). He was an outstanding physician and pharmacologist in the Ming Dynasty.

LI was well versed in Chinese materia medica and wrote a large number of works as famous *Bencao Gangmu* (《本草纲目》*Compendium of Materia Medica*). In addition, he also had a deep insight on meridians of TCM and wrote book *Qijing Bamai Kao* (《奇经八脉考》*A Study on the Eight Extra Meridians*) with one volume in 1572 A.D. This book collects different theories of various academic schools. Being concise and to the point, it is also methodical in the arrangement of all the chapters. It not only puts the running courses of the Eight Extra Meridians in order, but also expounds their functions and basic clinical manifestations of many problems, establishing an initial model about the diagnosis and treatment of extra-meridian conditions according to syndrome identification. *Qijing Bamai Kao* is a valuable literature data for studying the Eight Extra Meridians and is also a great contribution to the theory of meridian-collaterals.

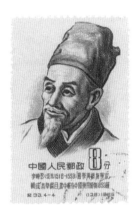

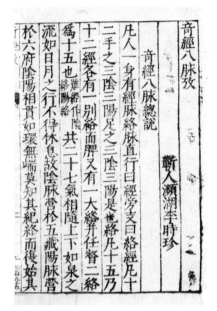

◇李时珍邮票

中国古代科学家邮票，1956年1月雕刻版，周建杨教授藏

A stamp for memorizing LI Shi-zhen
Stamp for memorizing Chinese ancient scientists, the engraved version of January of 1956, collected by Prof. ZHOU Jian-yang

◇《奇经八脉考》书影

明万历重刻本，中国中医科学院图书馆藏

Photograph of *Qijing Bamai Kao*
Re-printed version of Wanli regime of the Ming Dynasty, collected by the Library of CACMS

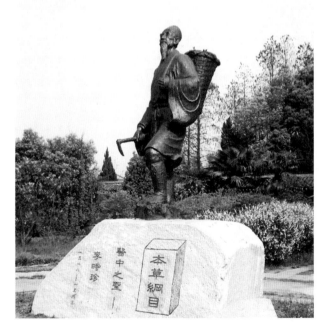

◇李时珍雕塑

位于湖北省蕲春县李时珍陵园

LI Shi-zhen's sculpture
Taken from LI Shi-zhen's Cemetery in Qichun County of Hubei Province

## 李时珍与《本草纲目》

李时珍家族世代业医,祖父是"铃医",父亲也是当地名医。李时珍自幼多病,三次考举人未中,后随父习医,成为当地名医。

公元1551年李时珍因治好了富顺王朱厚焜儿子的病而医名大显,被武昌的楚王聘为王府的"奉祠正",兼管良医所事务。之后,李时珍被推荐到太医院工作,授"太医院判"职务。期间,他饱览了王府和皇家珍藏的丰富典籍,看到了许多平时难以得见的药物标本,丰富了医学知识。但他淡于功名利禄,在太医院任职未及一年,便辞职归家,专心著述,于1578年撰成医药学巨著《本草纲目》,闻名海内外,达尔文称赞它是"中国古代的百科全书"。

## LI Shi-zhen and Bencao Gangmu

Li Shizhen was from a family of medicine for generations, his grandfather was a "bell doctor" and his father was a famous local physician. As a child, LI Shi-zhen was often ill. He failed three times in passing the imperial candidate examinations. Later he learned medicine from his father and became a well known regional physician.

In 1551 A.D., LI Shi-zhen became famous for curing the son of ZHU Hou-kun, the king of Fushun, and was appointed by the king of Chu in Wuchang as "an official in charge of ceremony honoring ancestors and medical affairs" in the palace. After that, LI Shi-zhen was recommended to work in the Imperial Academy of Medicine and appointed a post "medical administration". During this period, he had a chance to read valuable royal collection of rich classics and see precious drugs, which had enriched his medical knowledge.

However he was indifferent to fame and profit, so he resigned and returned home, devoting himself to writing. In 1578 A.D., he accomplished the great medical book *Bencao Gangmu* famous at home and abroad. Darwin regarded it as "an Encyclopedia of ancient China".

# 52

## 杨继洲与《针灸大成》
## YANG Ji-zhou and *Zhenjiu Dacheng* (*Great Compendium on Acupuncture and Moxibustion*)

杨继洲（约 1522—1620 年），又名济时，三衢（今浙江省衢州市）人，明代著名针灸医家。他出生医学世家，历任楚王府良医、太医院御医，以三针刺治愈山西巡抚御史赵文炳痿痹而名扬朝野。

杨继洲参考各书，编成《卫生针灸玄机秘要》3 卷，后由靳贤在此基础上补辑重编而成《针灸大成》10 卷，被尊为针灸经典。该书内容丰富，独具心得，吸取了明以前关于针灸学说的精华部分，搜集了当时民间流行的治疗方法，并增注歌赋，是继高武《针灸聚英》以后的又一次关于针灸文献的汇集，是一部翻印次数最多、流传最广的针灸专著，对后世针灸学产生了极其深远的影响。

YANG Ji-zhou (1522–1620 A.D.), also named Jishi, a native of Sanqu (current Quzhou City, Zhejiang Province), was a famous acupuncturist of the Ming Dynasty. He came from a long line of physicians, and was a highly qualified physician of Prince Chu Mansion and the imperial medical academy. He was famous in and outside the imperial court due to successfully curing ZHAO Wenbing's (the imperial circuit censor of Shanxi) flaccidity arthralgia by three acupuncture needles.

YANG compiled *Weisheng Zhenjiu Xuanji Miyao* (《卫生针灸玄机秘要》*Mysterious Essentials of Acupuncture-Moxibustion for Health Protection*) with 3 volumes in reference of various medical literature, upon which JIN Xian made a supplement and re-compiled the book *Zhenjiu Dacheng* (《针灸大成》 *Great Compendium on Acupuncture and Moxibustion*) containing 10 volumes. The *Zhenjiu Dacheng* was handed down for generations and regarded as an acupuncture classic. This book is very informative, not only imbibes essentials of acupuncture and moxibustion before the Ming Dynasty but also contains many new therapeutic methods and odes from the folk at that time, gathering all literature together for another time since the completion of GAO Wu's *Zhenjiu Juying*. This book, a monograph on acupuncture and moxibustion, has been reprinted again and again, and widely spread all over China with a far-reaching impact on the development of acupuncture and moxibustion for later generations.

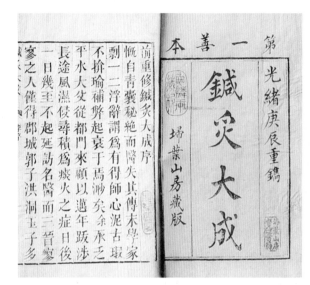

◇《针灸大成》书影
清刊本，中国中医科学院针灸研究所针灸博物馆藏

Photograph of *Zhenjiu Dacheng*
Block-printed version of the Qing Dynasty, collected by Chinese Museum of Acupuncture and Moxibustion, Institute of Acupuncture and Moxibustion, CACMS

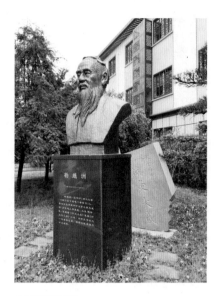

◇杨继洲雕塑
摄于浙江省衢州原衢江区中医院

YANG Ji-zhou's sculpture
Taken at the former Qujiang District Hospital of TCM, Quzhou City of Zhejiang Province

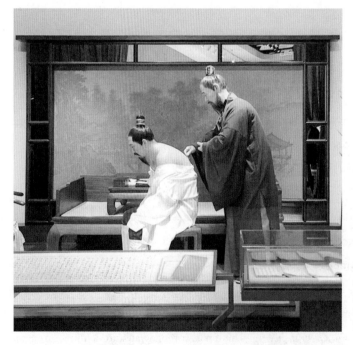

◇杨继洲三针治愈赵文炳痿痹复原场景
摄于浙江省衢州杨继洲针灸博物馆

The scene of Yang Jizhou's successfully treating ZHAO Wen-bing's flaccidity arthralgia by three acupuncture needles
Taken in the Museum of YANG Ji-zhou Acupuncture Hospital, Quzhou City of Zhejiang Province

## 《针灸大成》付梓

　　杨继洲行医 40 多年,临床经验丰富,尤精于针灸。家中藏有许多珍秘古籍,他从医后常常研读,得其真谛,遂汇同考异,亲自编纂,汇成一部针灸专著《卫生针灸玄机秘要》,共 3 卷,但未能刻成问世。后赵文炳帮助他将此书付梓出版,并委托晋阳人靳贤进行选集校正。杨继洲以诸家未备,广求群书,并将其中针灸内容一一摘录下来,汇集历代经典著作及当时诸家的精华,由靳贤为之补辑校注重编,命名为《针灸大成》。

## Publication of Zhenjiu Dacheng

　　YANG Ji-zhou had been practicing medicine for more than 40 years, and had rich clinical experience, especially in acupuncture. There were many rare ancient books in his family. He often studied them during his medical practice and learned the essence and got their true meaning. Then he combined the same or different textual research with his own compilation to form a monograph on acupuncture and moxibustion, *Weisheng Zhenjiu Xuanji Miyao* with 3 volumes but could not be published. Afterwards ZHAO Wen-bing entrusted JIN Xian, a native of Jinyang with collection and revision of the book and had it published.

　　Based on various medical literature and experience of physicians in the successive dynasties, YANG Ji-zhou collected and recorded the content related to acupuncture and moxibustion one by one, upon which JIN Xian made a supplement and re-compiled the book with the name of *Zhenjiu Dacheng*.

# 53

## 吴崑与《针方六集》

### WU Kun and *Zhenfang Liuji* (*Six Volumes of Acupuncture Prescriptions*)

吴崑（公元 1552—约 1620 年），字山甫，号鹤皋，安徽歙县人，明代针灸医家。

吴崑早年专攻经史子集，后弃儒学医，钻研岐黄之术，晚年致力著述，于明万历四十六年（公元 1618 年），撰成《针方六集》6 卷。该书选集类编诸家针灸文献，并辅以己见，发挥考证而成一家之言，内容包括腧穴、刺法、经论、针灸歌赋等，类分为 6 集，是一部汇集前人针灸理论和实践的针灸专著。

WU Kun (1552–about 1620 A.D.), courtesy name Shanfu and alias Hegao, a native of She County of Anhui Province, was a well-known acupuncturist in the Ming Dynasty.

Early in his career, WU majored in *Classics, History, Philosophers, Literary Collection* (four divisions of Chinese bibliography). Afterwards, he gave up learning of Confucianism and made great efforts in learning medicine and delving into herbal medicines. In his later years, he devoted himself to writing books. In the 46th year of Wanli regime (1618 A.D.) of the Ming Dynasty, he completed *Zhenfang Liuji* (《针方六集》*Six Volumes of Acupuncture Prescriptions*). This book collects various academic schools' documents on acupuncture and moxibustion and supplements the author's own viewpoints and research results, forming a distinctive doctrine. Its six volumes contain acupoints, needling techniques, meridian theory, odes of acupuncture and moxibustion, etc. It is a monograph on acupuncture and moxibustion theories and clinical experience of the predecessors.

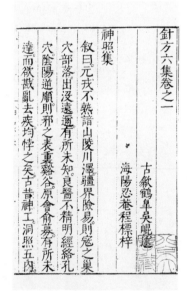

◇《针方六集》书影

明万历本，北京大学图书馆藏

Photograph of book *Zhenfang Liuji*
The edition of Wanli regime of the Ming Dynasty, collected by the Beijing University Library

# 54

# 张介宾与《类经图翼》
ZHANG Jie-bin and *Leijing Tuyi* (*Illustrated Supplementary to the Classified Canon*)

张介宾，字会卿，号景岳，又号通一子，山阴（浙江绍兴）人，约生于明嘉靖四十二年（公元 1563 年），卒于明崇祯十三年（公元 1640 年），明代著名医家。

张介宾天性颖慧，勤于读书，融会贯通百家之说，编成《类经》一书，并作《类经图翼》，以佐诠释，对《内经》的针灸理论有所发挥，贡献很大。《类经图翼》撰于明天启四年（公元 1624 年），共 11 卷，其中第 3~11 卷为针灸内容，插图很多，在每一穴下广泛征引诸家之说，条理清晰。此外，张氏另编有《类经附翼》4 卷，其中第 4 卷专录针灸歌赋。晚年又著《景岳全书》，为理法方药兼备之巨著，为后世医家所推崇。

ZHANG Jie-bin, courtesy name Huiqing, alias Jingyue and Tongyizi, a native of Shanyin (current Shaoxing of Zhejiang Province), was born in the 42$^{nd}$ year of Jiajing regime of the Ming Dynasty (1563 A.D.) and died in the 13$^{th}$ year of Chongzhen regime (1640 A.D.). He was a notable medical specialist of the Ming Dynasty.

ZHANG was very talented and wise in nature. He was diligent in reading, and thus assimilated a variety of theories of hundreds of academic schools to complete book *Leijing* (《类经》*Classified Canon*) and *Leijing Tuyi* (《类经图翼》*Illustrated Supplementary to the Classified Canon*) for annotating *Lei Jing*. These two books develop the academic theory of acupuncture and moxibustion of *Huangdi Neijing*. *Leijing Tuyi*, containing 11 volumes, was finished in the 4$^{th}$ year of Tianqi Age of the Ming Dynasty (1624 A.D.). Of the 11 volumes, 9 (3–11 volumes) focus on acupuncture and moxibustion, including many illustrations. In the legend of the illustrations, each acupoint follows multiple items of cited explanations of various academic schools, being well organized. In addition, ZHANG also edited additional *Leijing Fuyi* (《类经附翼》*Supplementary to the Classified Canon*) with 4 volumes, and specially containing songs and verses of acupuncture and moxibustion in the 4$^{th}$ Chapter. In his late years, he wrote *Jingyue Quanshu* (《景岳全书》*Jingyue's Complete Works*), a monumental works covering the theories, principles, prescriptions and materia medica, for which he was greatly canonized by the medical specialists in the later generations.

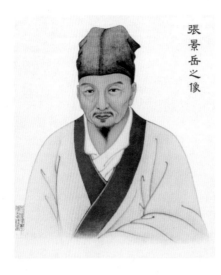

◇张景岳画像

　宋大仁绘

ZHANG Jing-yue's portrait
Drawn by SONG Da-ren

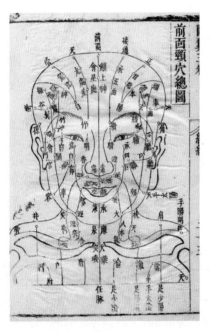
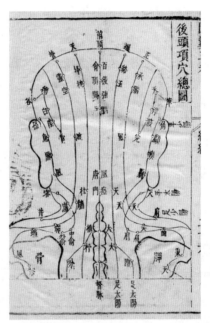

◇《类经图翼》书影

　明刻本，中国中医科学院图书馆藏

Photograph of *Leijing Tuyi*
A block-printed edition of the Ming Dynasty, collected by the Library of CACMS

**张景岳妙法逐铁钉**

相传，一户王姓人家有一儿子，刚满一岁。一天，其母随手拿一枚铁钉给他玩，小儿误塞入口，吞到喉间出不来。其母见状，倒提小孩两足，想倒出铁钉，小儿反而鼻孔喷血，情况非常危急，小儿的父亲号呼求救。恰好张景岳路过，急命其母将小儿抱正，小儿"哇"地一声哭开了，景岳断定铁钉已入肠胃。

张景岳根据《神农本草经》上"铁畏朴硝"的记载，想出一个治疗方案。他取来活磁石一钱、朴硝二钱，研为细末，用熟猪油、蜂蜜调好，让小儿服下。不久，小儿解下一物，大如芋子，润滑无棱，拨开一看，里面正好裹着那枚误吞下的铁钉。小儿父母感激不已，请教其中奥秘。景岳解释说：所用四药互有联系，朴硝若没有吸铁的磁石就不能附在钉上；磁石若没有泻下的朴硝就不能逐出铁钉；猪油、蜂蜜润滑肠道，使铁钉易于排出；四药同功合力，裹护铁钉从肠道排出。

# Zhang Jingyue's magic way of taking out the nail

According to legend, a WANG family had a son who was just over one year old. One day, his mother took an iron nail to play with him, and the child put the nail into his mouth by mistake and swallowed it in the throat. The mother saw the situation, inverted the child's feet, wanted to pour out the nail, but the child started to have nasal bleeding. The case was very urgent. The father of the child called for help. When the accident happened, ZHANG Jing-yue just passed by. He asked urgently the mother to hold the child in her arms. "Wow", the child cried loudly. Jingyue was sure that the nail had entered his stomach.

According to the records of "iron being antagonistic to Po Xiao (朴硝 Crude Mirabilite, Sodium Sulphate)" in *Shennong Bencao Jing*, ZHANG Jing-yue came up with an idea for the treatment. He took about 3g of alive Ci Shi (磁石 Magnetite) and 6g of Po Xiao (朴硝 Crude Mirabilite), and ground them into fine powder mixed with cooked lard and honey and let the child to take. Soon, the child had bowel movement, feces excreted was as big as a taro, smooth without edges. When it was opened, the right nail was found. The parents were so grateful and asked for the secret of the treatment. Jing-yue explained that the four drugs used were related to each other. Without attracted Ci Shi, Po Xiao would not be attached to the nail; without purgative Po Xiao, Ci Shi would not be able to remove the nail; lard and honey could moisten the intestine, so that the nail could be easily discharged. The joint actions of the four drugs made it possible that the protected wrapped nail could be excreted from the intestine.

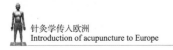

# 55

## 针灸学传入欧洲
## Introduction of acupuncture to Europe

大约 14 世纪,意大利著名旅行家马可波罗在一封信中谈到中国医疗用的针。16 世纪时,欧洲已有关于应用针术的记载。大约 17 世纪,法国一位天主教士 Du. Helbe 对中国针灸医学作了介绍,并绘有各穴道图表。公元 1658 年,丹麦人旁特(Dane Jacob Bondt)在印度自然史和医学的书中,记述了当地医生采用针术治病情况。这个时期,针灸代表性著作有荷兰瑞尼(Wilbelmi Ten Rhyne)的《论针刺术:风湿病的治疗》,德国哥荷马(Gehema J.A.)的《应用中国灸术治疗痛风》和法国萨朗弟爱的《电针》。17 世纪末,德国医生还将中国针灸术介绍到法国。18 世纪以后,针灸通过传教士或医生分别传到了法国、英国和意大利等欧洲国家。

As early as in the 14th century, Marco Polo, a well-known Italian traveler, mentioned Chinese acupuncture needle in one of his letters. In the 16th century, records about application of acupuncture techniques appeared in Europe. In about the 17th century, Catholic Priest Du. Helbe from France made an introduction about Chinese acupuncture medicine and drew some diagrams of different acupoints. In 1658 A.D., Dane Jacob Bondt described how local doctors applied needling therapy to treatment of some disorders in books of Indian natural history and medicine. During this period, the representative works on acupuncture were *On Acupuncture Techniques*: *Treatment of Rheumatism* written by Wilbelmi Ten Rhyne from Netherlands, *Application of Chinese Moxibustion to Treatment of Arthrolithiasis* written by Gehema J.A. from Germany, and *Electroacupuncture* written by Gean Baptiste Sarlandiere from France. At the end of 17th century, Chinese acupuncture was introduced to France by German doctors. After the 18th century, acupuncture was spread to more European countries as France, Britain, Italy, etc. either by preachers or medical practitioners.

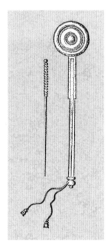

◇《论针刺术：风湿病的治疗》扉页及针具插图

Flyleaf and illustration of acupuncture needles in book
*On Acupuncture Techniques: Treatment of Rheumatism*

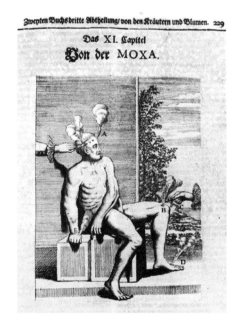

◇瓦伦提尼（Valentini M.B.）专著中的灸法图

Illustration of Moxibustion in Valentini M.B.'s monograph

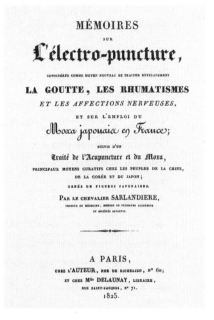

◇萨朗弟爱的电针（刺）疗法著作扉页

Flyleaf of *Electroacupuncture* written by Gean Baptiste Sarlandiere

### 欧洲较早的针灸专著

1676 年,荷兰人布绍夫(Hermann Busschof)介绍中国针灸术的文稿被译成英文,取名《痛风论文集》,在伦敦出版,创用了 Moxibustion 一词。同年,德国人吉尔弗西斯(Geilfusius, R.W.)用德文撰写《灸术》一书介绍灸法,在德国马尔堡出版。

荷兰人瑞尼(Wilbelm Ten Rhyne)医生,在日本和爪哇期间接触到针灸术并将其介绍到了欧洲,于 1683 年在伦敦出版了《论针刺术:风湿病的治疗》一书,这是西方较早系统介绍针刺术的专著,"针刺"翻译为 Acupunctura,就是通过该书在西方语言中得以固定,书中附有针具图一幅。同年,德国人哥荷马(Gehema J.A.)在汉堡出版了《应用中国灸术治疗痛风》一书,提出灸法是治疗痛风最迅速、最适合、最安全的疗法;公元 1686 年德国医学教授瓦伦提尼(Valentini M.B.)在荷兰莱顿市出版的专著 Historiae Moxae cum adjunctis medicationibus Podagrae 中介绍了采用灸法配合药物治疗痛风,书中将灸术描述为:无痛的有效疗法,尤其是对痛风、关节炎等。

1825 年,法国医学博士萨朗弟爱(Sarlandière)以法文撰写了第一部关于电针(刺)疗法的著作,介绍在法国采用针灸疗法治疗痛风、风湿和神经系统的著作,这是现存最早关于用电针治病的记载。1863 年,法国驻华领事达布理(Dabry P.)出版《中国医学大全》一书,节译了杨继洲的《针灸大成》,成为当时法国针灸师的案头读物,对法国针灸界影响较大。

## Earlier acupuncture-moxibustion monographs in Europe

In 1676 A.D., a manuscript about Chinese acupuncture and moxibustion presented by Hermann Busschof of the Netherlands was translated into English and published in London with the name of *Collection of Treatises on Gout*, in which the term Moxibustion was initiated. In the same year, German Geilfusius (R.W.) wrote a book *Moxibustion* in German, which was published in Marburg, Germany.

Dr.Wilbelm Ten Rhyne of the Netherlands, who came into contact with acupuncture during his stay in Japan and Java, introduced acupuncture to Europe. In 1683 A.D., the book *On Acupuncture Techniques: Treatment of Rheumatism* was published in London, which was regarded as a systematic acupuncture monograph introduced early in Europe. The Chinese "针刺" (Zhen Ci) was translated as "Acupunctura" and fixed in Western language. Attached to the book, there was a picture of needles.

In the same year, Gehema J.A. of Germany published the book *Application of Chinese Moxibustion to Treatment of Arthrolithiasis* in Hamburg and proposed that moxibustion had been the most proper and safe treatment with quickest effect for gout; in 1686, German medical professor Valentini M.B. published a monograph *Historiae Moxae cum adjunctis medicationibus Podagrae* in Leiden, the Netherlands, in which combination of medication with moxibustion was introduced and moxibustion was described as a painless and effective therapy, especially for treatment of gout and arthritis.

In 1825 A.D., Sarlandiere, a French doctor of medicine, wrote the first book on Electro-acupuncture (acupuncture) in French, introducing the use of acupuncture in the treatment of gout, rheumatism and diseases of the nerve system in France, which has been the earliest extant record of electro-acupuncture. In 1863 A.D., Dabry P., the French Consul in China published *Zhongguo Yixue Daquan* (《中国医学大全》*A Complete Manual of Chinese Medicine*) by translating parts of Yang Jizhou's *Zhenjiu Dacheng* which became a desk book for French acupuncturists at that time and had exerted a great influence on French acupuncture and moxibustion circles.

# 56

## 吴谦与《医宗金鉴》
## WU Qian and *Yizong Jinjian* (*Golden Mirror of Medicine*)

吴谦,字六吉,安徽歙县人,约生于清康熙二十八年(公元 1689 年),卒于乾隆二十四年(公元 1759 年),清代名医。

吴谦曾任清廷御医,官至太医院判。乾隆四年,他奉敕开始编纂大型综合性医书,于乾隆七年(公元 1742 年)编撰成《医宗金鉴》90 卷。其中第 79~86 卷是《刺灸心法要诀》,内容包括经络、腧穴、针灸证治及刺灸法部,其基本形式为歌诀及注文两个层次,歌诀多直接抄自前代文献或据他书原文改编而成,注文部分反映了编者的学术见解。该书首次强调了经络图与经穴图的不同性质,为后人正确把握二者间的关系提供了重要启示。该书刊刻精良,内容较为浅显,对清代的针灸学产生了深远影响。

WU Qian, Liuji in courtesy name, a native of She County of Anhui Province, was born in the 28th year of Kangxi regime (1689 A.D.) of the Qing Dynasty, and died in the 24th year of Qianlong regime (1759 A.D.). He was a well-known physician during the Emperor Yongzheng and Emperor Qianlong ages.

As an official of the Imperial Academy of Medicine serving the inner court, WU was appointed to be the primary one of the two general organizers to compile large comprehensive medical book in the 4th year of Qianlong Age. In the 7th year (1742 A.D.), they finished *Yizong Jinjian* (《医宗金鉴》*Golden Mirror of Medicine*) embracing 90 volumes. Of the 90 volumes, the 79th to 86th are referred to *Cijiu Xinfa Yaojue* (《刺灸心法要诀》*Essentials of Acupuncture and Moxibustion in Verse*), covering meridian-collaterals, acupoints, clinical indications and treatment, and needling-moxibustion techniques which were written in two forms of verses and annotations. The verses are directly quoted or edited from previous generations' literature or original texts of other writers, and the annotation part expounds WU's own academic views. The book *Yizong Jinjian* for the first time emphasizes the different characteristics of meridian-collateral diagram and acupoint diagram, providing an important enlightenment for the descendants to correctly grasp their relationship. This book is excellent in printing and easy to understand in the contents, and plays a profound influence on acupuncture-moxibustion medicine in the Qing Dynasty.

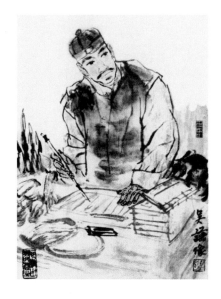

◇吴谦画像

　　引自《中国历代名医图传》（陈雪楼主编，江苏科学技术出版社，1987 年）

WU Qian's portrait

Cited from book *Zhongguo Lidai Mingyi Tuzhuan* (Editor-in-chief CHEN Xue-lou, published by Jiangsu Science and Technology Press in 1987)

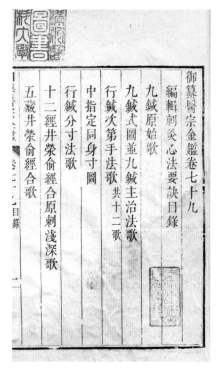

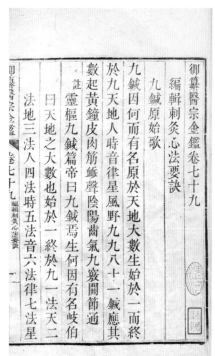

◇《医宗金鉴·刺灸心法要诀》书影

　　清乾隆七年壬戌（1742 年）湖南坊刻本，中国中医科学院图书馆藏

Photograph of *Yizong Jinjian: Cijiu Xinfa Yaojue*

Hunan workshop block-printed edition of the Qing Dynasty, the 7th year of Qianlong's Age (Renxu year, 1742 A.D.), collected by the Library of CACMS

# 57

# 李守先与《针灸易学》
## LI Shou-xian and *Zhenjiu Yixue* (*Acupuncture and Moxibustion Are Easy to Learn*)

　　《针灸易学》作者为李守先,字善述,河南长葛县人,生于乾隆元年(公元1736年),卒年不详,清代医家。

　　《针灸易学》撰于清嘉庆三年(公元1798年),分上下两卷。李氏认为学针灸"首学手法,次学认症,而以寻穴为末务",故全书分为"手法""认症""寻穴"三部分,重点介绍针灸方法及要穴的应用,记述十四经穴及奇穴。该书"将古法著之于前,愚见列之于后,浅而易知,显而易明",便于初学者习用,是一本重视针灸手法和针灸学知识普及的书籍。

　　LI Shou-xian, Shanshu in courtesy name, a man of Changge County of Henan Province, was born in the 1st year of Qianlong Age (1736 A.D.), but his death date was unclear. He was a physician of the Qing Dynasty.

　　LI wrote the book *Zhenjiu Yixue* (《针灸易学》*Acupuncture and Moxibustion Are Easy to Learn*) consisting of two volumes in the 3rd year of Jiaqing Age of the Qing Dynasty (1798 A.D.). He proposed that in learning acupuncture-moxibustion, one should go through three steps, acupuncture needle manipulation techniques the first, pattern identification (diagnosis) the second, and reasonable selection of acupoints the last. Thus, this book was written in the same order, focusing on the performing skills of acupuncture and moxibustion and flexible application of important acupoints, such as those of the 14 meridians and extra-meridians. In this book, "the predecessors' methods were introduced in the front part, followed by the LI's own methods, being easy to learn and concise in the content". It is a book laying stress on needling manipulations and popularization of basic acupuncture-moxibustion learnings, being suitable for the beginners.

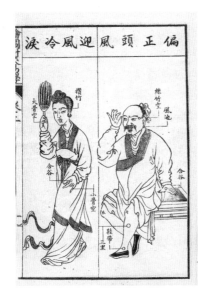
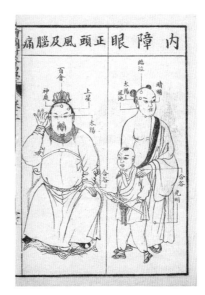

◇病症治疗图

　　引自《绘图针灸易学》，民国五年仲冬上海萃英书庄重校，中国中医科学院图书馆藏

A picture of clinical treatment

Cited from the book *Huitu Zhenjiu Yixue* (《绘图针灸易学》*Illustrated Book for Easily Learning Acupuncture and Moxibustion)*, re-revised by Shanghai Cuiying Book Store in the midwinter of the 5th year of Republic of China, collected by the Library of CACMS

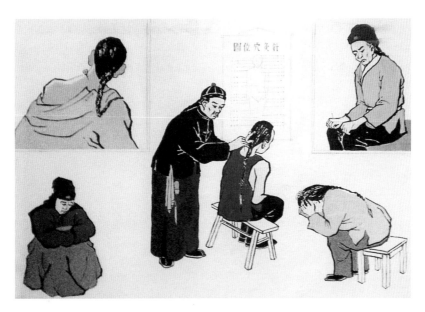

◇李守先针灸治疗疟疾

　　摄于湖南中医药大学针灸陈列馆

LI Shou-xian treating malaria with acupuncture and moxibustion

Taken in the Museum of Acupuncture and Moxibustion of Hunan University of TCM

**李守先针灸治疟**

　　李守先年少时就已经开始学习针灸,终日精勤不倦,但因无名师指点、传授,对自己成为一名杰出的针灸医生,缺乏信心,直到清乾隆年间的那次疟疾大流行才使他找回了自信。乾隆五十一年,疟疾盛行,十人之中有九人患疟疾,当时李守先已51岁。他选择那些年青体壮的疟疾患者,用针灸治疗,起先三人之中有一人获效,后来五人之中有三人获效,之后再阅读、研究针灸医书,并用于指导治疗疟疾,疗效大增。这一时期李守先用针灸治疗疟疾,前后共22天,有临床疗效的患者多达437人。

## Malaria treated with acupuncture and moxibustion by LI Shou-xian

　　LI Shou-xian started to learn acupuncture when he was young. He studied and worked hard all day. However, he lacked confidence in becoming an outstanding acupuncturist because he did not have a famous teacher for instruction and guidance. It was not until the occurrence of epidemic malaria in the reign of Emperor Qianlong of the Qing Dynasty did he regain his confidence. In the 51st year of Qianlong, malaria was prevalent. Nine of the ten people suffered from malaria. LI Shou-xian was 51 years old at that time. He chose those young and strong malaria patients and treated them with acupuncture. At first, one of the three patients was effectively treated, then three of the five patients were treated with effects. Consequently, he read and studied acupuncture books further and used the knowledge to guide the treatment of malaria. The curative effect was greatly increased. During that period within 22 days, LI Shou-xian treated 437 patients of malaria with acupuncture and achieved good clinical therapeutic results.

# 58

## 李学川与《针灸逢源》
LI Xue-chuan and *Zhenjiu Fengyuan* (*The Source of Acupuncture and Moxibustion*)

李学川,字三源,号邓尉山人,江苏吴县人,清代针灸名医,生卒年代不详。

至清代,针灸医学逐渐由兴盛走向衰退,李学川感慨当时轻视针灸的社会风气,于清嘉庆二十年(公元 1815 年),综合《灵枢》《素问》《针灸甲乙经》经穴的异同,结合自己的临证经验而著成《针灸逢源》6 卷。该书内容丰富,论述精辟,去诸医籍之弊,总结了清中期以前针灸医学的理论与实践,对后世针灸学发展产生了一定的影响。

LI Xue-chuan, Sanyuan in courtesy name and Dengwei Shanren (Hermit) in alias, a native of Wu County of Jiangsu Province, was a distinguished acupuncturist in the Qing Dynasty. His birthday and death day remain unknown.

Till the early period of the Qing Dynasty, acupuncture-moxibustion medicine had been declining gradually from prosperity to recession. In the 20th year of Jiaqing Age of the Qing Dynasty (1815 A.D.), ignoring the temporal ethos of neglecting acupuncture-moxibustion and combining his own clinical experience, LI Xue-chuan carefully studied the similarities and differences in textual descriptions about meridian acupoints in *Lingshu*, *Suwen*, and *Zhenjiu Jiayi Jing* to write the book *Zhenjiu Fengyuan* (《针灸逢源》*The Source of Acupuncture and Moxibustion*) with 6 volumes. This book summarized the theories and clinical experience on acupuncture and moxibustion accumulated in various historical periods prior to the middle stage of the Qing Dynasty. Being very informative and incisive in the discourse, it eliminates shortcomings of various medical books, inducing a certain impact on the development of acupuncture-moxibustion medicine in the later generations.

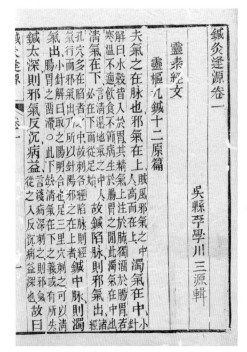

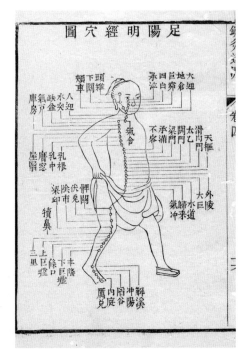

◇《针灸逢源》书影

清刻本，中国中医科学院图书馆藏

Photograph of *Zhenjiu Fengyuan*

Block-printed version of the Qing Dynasty, collected by the Library of CACMS

# 59

# 针灸术传入美国
Introduction of acupuncture-moxibustion to the U.S.

中国的针灸术大约在 19 世纪初,通过欧洲传入美国,美国医学杂志选载欧洲应用针刺术的经验和学术报告,开始认识针灸。1820 年,美国医学杂志《医学原创论文及情报信息库》发表题为《针刺疗法:对其治疗作用的思考》一文,然而美国医学界对此态度谨慎。1825 年,美国著名化学家、医生巴彻·弗兰克林(Franklin Bache)在费城翻译出版了法国莫兰德(Morand)《针刺术研究报告》(法文版)一书的英文版,并亲自选择病例在临床上试用针刺术治疗,这是现知由美国出版的最早针灸书。1830 年,塔列费罗(Taliaferro W.T.)在《美国医学科学杂志》上发表了"艾灸成功治疗瘫痪病例",这是美国早期文献中一篇关于灸法实际应用的报道。

Chinese acupuncture therapy was introduced from Europe to the U.S. in about early 19th century when European scholar's acupuncture experience and academic reports had been published in *The American Journals of the Medical Sciences (Am J Med Sci)*. Then, American people began to know acupuncture. In 1820, *Original Medical Thesis and Information Database*, a medical journal of America, published an essay titled *Acupuncture Therapy: Overview of its Therapeutic Effects*, but the American medical circle still remained cautious about it. In 1825, at Philadelphia, American chemist, Dr. Franklin Bache translated Morand's book *Memoire sur l'acupuncture duivi d'une serie d'observations recueillies sous les yeux de M* from French into English *Memoir on acupuncturation embracing a series of cases drawn up under the inspection of M. Julius Cloquet* which is known to be the earliest acupuncture publication in the U.S. In 1830, Taliaferro's article titled *Successful Treatment of Paralysis by Moxibustion* was published in Am J Med Sci, which is known to be the earliest report about practical application of moxibustion in the U.S.

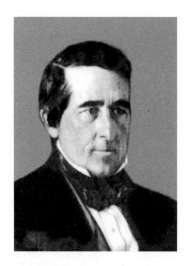

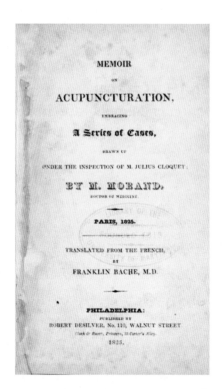

◇巴彻·弗兰克林肖像

　　引自巴彻·弗兰克林给罗伯特·黑尔的一封信(《化学历史》, 1994 )

Portrait of Franklin Bache, M.D.
Quoted from the Letter of Franklin Bache to Robert Hare (*Bull Hist Chem*, 1994)

◇《针刺术研究报告》扉页

　　法国莫兰德 ( Morand ) 著, 美国巴彻·弗兰克林 ( Franklin Bache ) 译, 马里兰大学图书馆藏

Flyleaf of book "*Memoir on acupuncture embracing a series of cases drawn up under the inspection of M. Julius Cloque*" (Philadelphia: Desilver, 1825 A.D.)
Written by Morand (France), translated by Franklin Bache (U.S.), preserved in the library of Maryland University

# 60

## 清代道光皇帝禁针诏
### Emperor Daoguang's edict for prohibiting acupuncture in the Qing Dynasty

针灸一科,自唐代在太医署设为专科以来,在历代太医院中,一直作为专科独立设置。直至清代道光皇帝在其继位第二年(公元 1822 年),颁布禁针诏,下令云:"针灸一法,由来已久,然以针刺火灸,究非奉君之所宜,太医院针灸一科,着永远停止。"虽然针灸在太医院中被禁止使用,但由于其疗效确切,操作简便,在民间仍然广泛应用。

Since the Tang Dynasty, acupuncture-moxibustion as a specialized subject, had been set up independently in the imperial medical academy. In the 2<sup>nd</sup> year of the Emperor Daoguang in the Qing Dynasty (1822 A.D.), he issued an edict for prohibiting acupuncture, saying that "the acupuncture and moxibustion therapies have a long history, but, both needling and moxibustion are definitely not suitable to serve the emperor. Thus, the subjects of acupuncture and moxibustion in the imperial medical academy should be prohibited forever from now on". Despite being prohibited in the imperial academy of medicine, these therapies were still employed widely in the civilian at that time due to its good efficacy and simple operation.

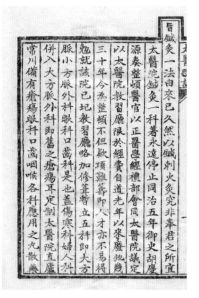

◇清道光皇帝禁针诏
　引自《太医院志》

Emperor Daoguang's edict for prohibiting acupuncture in the Qing Dynasty
Cited from the *Taiyiyuan Zhi* (《太医院志》*Records of the Imperial Academy of Medicine*)

# 61

## 针灸西传的代表人物苏理

George Soulié de Morant, a representative figure of acupuncture who introduced acupuncture to the Western countries

民国时期,法国是西方传播针灸最有影响的国家之一,对于针灸西传发挥了重要作用。把针灸带入法国的最有代表性的人物是苏理(George Soulié de Morant,公元 1878—1955 年)。

1901 年初,苏理来华工作,曾任法国驻上海领事。清光绪二十八年(公元 1902 年),北京地区霍乱流行,由于使用了针灸疗法,治愈率高达 60%。由此,苏理对针灸学产生了浓厚兴趣,向多位中医师学习针灸。1911 年 1 月,苏理回国,将针灸医术带回法国,后专门从事针灸医疗工作,因用针灸治疗哮喘有奇效而显名,极大地改善了法国针灸界之状况。他先后撰有一系列文章和针灸著作(如《中国针刺术》),向法国和欧洲传播针灸医学。因其在法国针灸界的卓越贡献,被尊称为法国"针灸之父"。

In the period of the Republic of China, France was one of the most powerful countries in regard of spreading acupuncture therapy in the West. George Soulié de Morant (1878–1955 A.D.) is the representative figure who introduced acupuncture therapy to France.

At the beginning of 1901 A.D., Soulié de Morant came to China and was once appointed to be French Consul of Shanghai. In the 28th year of Guangxu Age of the Qing Dynasty (1902 A.D.), cholera was epidemic in Beijing region. However, the cure rate was 60%, thanks to acupuncture and moxibustion therapy. It was thus that Soulié de Morant became interested in acupuncture learnings, and studied it from several physicians of TCM. In January of 1911 A.D., Soulié de Morant returned and brought acupuncture skills back to France. Later on, he began to exclusively engage in acupuncture work, became famous due to his

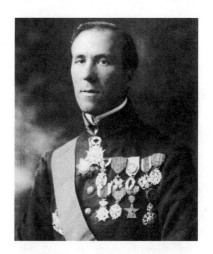

◇苏理像
摄于云南省中医药民族医药博物馆中医西传分馆

George Soulié de Morant's portrait
Taken at the Branch Hall for Introducing TCM to the West, Yunnan Museum of TCM and Ethnomedicine

wonderful therapeutic effect in the treatment of asthma, which greatly improved the condition of French acupuncture circle. He wrote a series of articles and books, such as *Précis de la vrai Acuponcture Chinoise* (*Chinese Acupuncture*), etc. which were spread widely in France and Europe. Owing to his distinguished contribution to French acupuncture, he was respected to be the "father of French acupuncture".

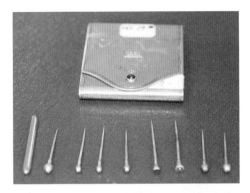

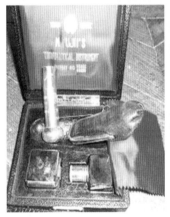
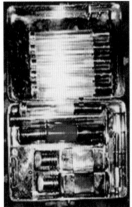
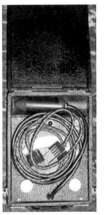
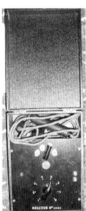

◇苏理使用的金针、器械包和电针仪
摄于云南省中医药民族医药博物馆中医西传分馆

Gold needle, toolkit and electroacupuncture apparatus used by George Soulié de Morant
Taken at the Branch Hall for Introducing TCM to the West, Yunnan Museum of TCM and Ethnomedicine

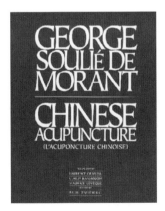

◇《中国针刺术》封面

The cover page of *Précis de la vrai Acuponcture Chinoise* (*Chinese Acupuncture*)

# 62

# 近代针灸学家承澹盦

## CHENG Dan-an, a well-known acupuncture expert in modern times

承澹盦（淡安）（1899—1957 年），又名启桐，江苏江阴市华墅人，民国及中华人民共和国初期著名的针灸医家及中医教育家。1929 年，他创办最早的针灸函授教育——中国针灸学研究社。1933 年 10 月，创办最早的针灸学术刊物——《针灸杂志》。1954 年，任江苏省中医进修学校（南京中医药大学的前身）首任校长，为中国科学院学部委员。他培养的学员遍及海内外，为我国针灸事业的振兴和针灸走向世界做出了卓越贡献。其主要著作有《中国针灸治疗学》《中国针灸学讲义》《中国针灸学》《校注十四经发挥》等，其中《中国针灸治疗学》是最具有代表性的一部针灸专著。

Mr. CHENG Dan-an (1899–1957), also named Qi-tong, was from Jiangyin Huashu of Jiangsu Province. He was a well-known acupuncture expert and an educator of TCM in the Republic of China and in the early period of the People's Republic of China (P.R. China).

In 1929, Mr. CHENG founded the Research Society of Chinese Acupuncture and Moxibustion, the earliest acupuncture and moxibustion correspondence course in China. In October of 1933, he set up *Journal of Acupuncture and Moxibustion* (《针灸杂志》), the earliest academic publication on acupuncture and moxibustion. In 1954, Mr. CHENG was appointed to be the first president of Jiangsu Provincial Training School of TCM (the predecessor of Nanjing University of TCM) and the member of Chinese Academy of Sciences. His students distribute everywhere in China and in many foreign countries. He made a remarkable contribution to the development of acupuncture-moxibustion cause and its globalwide spread. The books he wrote include *Zhongguo Zhenjiu Zhiliao Xue* (《中国针灸治疗学》*Chinese Acupuncture and Moxibustion Therapeutics*), *Zhongguo Zhenjiuxue Jiangyi* (《中国针灸学讲义》*Teaching Material for Chinese Acupuncture and Moxibustion*), *Zhongguo Zhenjiu Xue* (《中国针灸学》*Chinese Acupuncture and Moxibustion*), and *Jiaozhu Shisi Jing Fahui* (《校注十四经发挥》*Revised and Annotated Elucidation of the Fourteen Meridians*), among which *Zhongguo Zhenjiu Zhiliao Xue* is his most representative monograph.

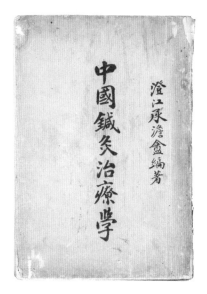

◇《中国针灸治疗学》封面

1931 年铅印本

中国中医科学院针灸研究所针灸博物馆藏

The cover page of *Zhongguo Zhenjiu Zhiliao Xue*
Lead-printed version in 1931, collected by Chinese Museum of Acupuncture
and Moxibustion, Institute of Acupuncture and Moxibustion, CACMS

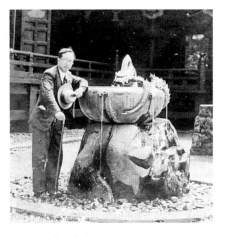

◇承淡盦赴日考察留影

摄于东京（1934 年），承淡盦故居藏

Mr. CHENG Dan-an in Japan
Taken in 1934, preserved in CHENG Dan-an's
former residence, Tokyo

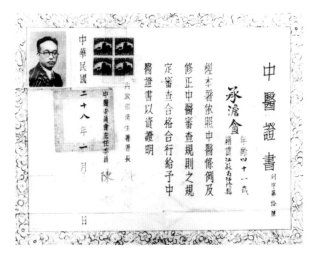

◇承淡盦中医证书

1939 年（民国二十八年）颁发

TCM Certificate of Mr. CHENG Dan-an
Issued at the 28th year of the Republic of China, in 1939

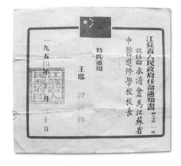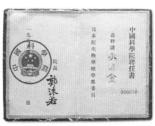

◇承淡盦的部分证件

摄于江苏省苏州市承淡盦故居

Licenses and certificates of Mr. CHENG Dan-an
Taken in CHENG Dan-an's former residence
in Suzhou of Jiangsu Province

# 63

# 中国针灸学研究社
## Research Society of Chinese Acupuncture and Moxibustion

1929 年,承澹盦在江苏吴县望亭创办了近代中医教育史上最早的针灸函授机构——"中国针灸学研究社",招收全国各地学员,以寄发针灸教学材料和函询解答问题为主的通信函授方式培养针灸人才。两年后因经费绌窘停办。1932 年 10 月,该社迁无锡市重建,先后开辟教学实验场所和实习科。1934 年,研究社组织结构更趋完备,初具专业学校规模。

1935 年,承澹盦在研究社的基础上创办了近代中国的针灸专门学校——"中国针灸学讲习所"。1937 年 2 月,讲习所更名为"中国针灸医学专门学校",后因战争爆发,承澹盦又辗转于皖、赣、湘、鄂、川等地开办学习班或分校。抗战胜利后,承澹盦返回故里,其时国事日非,民不聊生,研究社被迫中辍。中华人民共和国成立后,承澹盦受到极大鼓舞,中国针灸学研究社于 1951 年在苏州恢复社业。

In 1929, Mr. CHENG Dan-an founded the "Research Society of Chinese Acupuncture and Moxibustion" (RSCAM) in Wangting of Wu County of Jiangsu Province, the earliest correspondence course institution of acupuncture and moxibustion in modern education history of TCM. This institution accepted students from every part of China to cultivate professionals for acupuncture and moxibustion by sending them teaching materials, explaining and answering questions via correspondences, but it was closed down two years later due to budget shortage. In October 1932, this institute was re-established and moved to Wuxi City, and successively started teaching experimental workshops and clinical practice workshops. Until 1934 the organization structure became complete and processed the size of a primary professional training school.

In 1935, Mr. CHENG set up a "Workshop of Chinese Acupuncture and Moxibustion", a modern speciality school on the basis of his "Research Society". In February of 1937, this Workshop was renamed "Chinese Technical School of Acupuncture and Moxibustion". After the outbreak of Anti-Japanese War, Mr. CHENG was forced to shift to Anhui, Jiangxi, Hunan, Hubei, Sichuan provinces, and other places of China in succession, where he opened special training classes or branch schools.

After the victory of Anti-Japanese War, Mr. CHENG went back to his homeland, when, China was in ruins, people had no means to live, and his research society was forced to be closed. After founding of the People's Republic of China, Mr. CHENG was greatly inspired and re-opened the "RSCAM" in 1951 in Suzhou City.

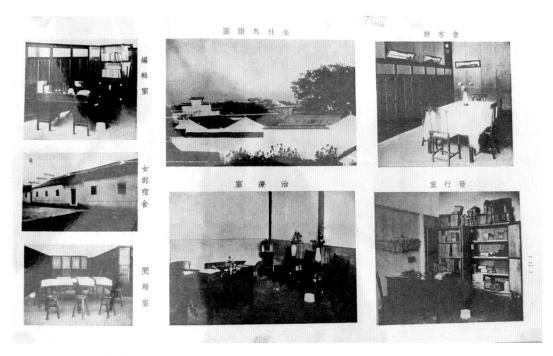

◇中国针灸学研究社掠影

Scenery of the RSCAM

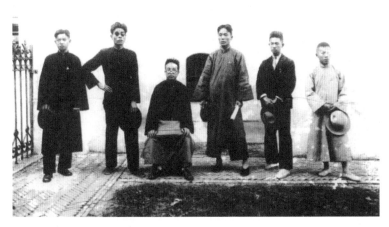

◇中国针灸学研究社实习生第一届毕业合影（1932年）

A group photo of first graduates of the first session of RSCAM (1932)

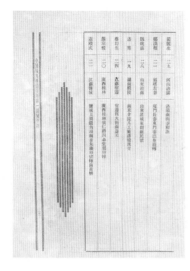
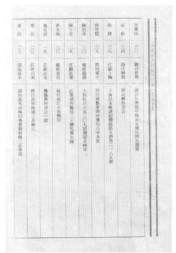
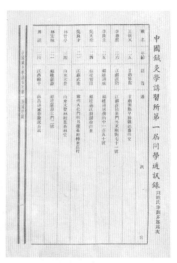

◇中国针灸学讲习所第一届同学通讯录

引自《针灸杂志》,第 3 卷第 1 期（1936 年）

Address list of students of the first session of the Workshop of Chinese Acupuncture and Moxibustion
Cited from *Journal of Acupuncture and Moxibustion*, 1936, 3 (1)

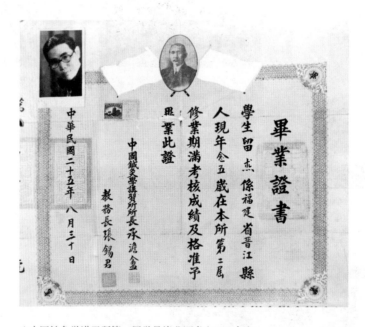

◇中国针灸学讲习所第二届学员毕业证书（1936 年）

摄于湖南中医药大学针灸陈列馆

Graduation certificate of students from the second session of the Workshop of
Chinese Acupuncture and Moxibustion (1936)
Taken at the acupuncture exhibition hall, Hunan University of TCM

**最早的针灸杂志**

　　承澹盦先生在开办"中国针灸学研究社"期间,为方便学员交流学术经验,于1933 年创办了近代中医历史上最早的针灸专业杂志——《针灸杂志》。内容辟有"论文""专载""杂著""问答""社友成绩栏"和"医讯"等专栏,原为双月刊,后改为月刊,至抗日战争共出版 36 期,抗战后复刊出版 6 期,后改名为《针灸医学》,出版了 15 期。

## *The earliest acupuncture and moxibustion journal*

　　In 1933, during the period of founding of the Research Society of Chinese Acupuncture and Moxibustion, Mr. CHENG Dan-an established *Journal of Acupuncture and Moxibustion*, the earliest academic publication on acupuncture and moxibustion in the history of modern Chinese medicine with the columns of "papers", "spacial topics", "miscellaneous works", "questions and answers", "achievements of community members" and "medical news" in order to promote the academic exchanges of experience among the medical doctors and students. The former was a bimonthly journal, then changed into a monthly one. Till the Anti-Japanese War, a total of 36 issues had been published. After the Anti-Japanese War, 6 resumed publications were distributed, and then the journal was renamed *Acupuncture and Moxibustion Medicine*, another 15 issues were published.

# 64

# 针坛优秀女性朱琏

## ZHU Lian, an outstanding woman in the acupuncture field

朱琏（1909—1978年），字景雩，原籍安徽，生于江苏溧阳。朱琏是一位现当代针灸发展史上的卓越女性，在针灸科研、教育、理论、临床、国际交流等方面均做出重大贡献。1951年3月，出版其专著《新针灸学》，被称为"运用现代科学观点与方法，探索提高针灸技术与科学原理的第一部重要著作"，被译成朝、俄、越等多种文字出版。新中国成立后，她创建了中央人民政府卫生部针灸疗法实验所（今中国中医科学院针灸研究所）并任所长。

她总结的"缓慢捻进法"，已形成独具特色的"广西针灸流派"针法（也称"朱琏针法"）；首创的"艾卷悬起灸"及发明的"埋针"技术，成为当今针灸临床常用之方法。

Ms. ZHU Lian (1909–1978), Jingyu in courtesy name, was born in Liyang of Jiangsu Province with her ancestral home in Anhui Province. She was an outstanding female leader in modern and contemporary China in the development of history of acupuncture-moxibustion, and made a great contribution to the acupuncture research, education, theoretical study, clinical practice, international exchange, etc. In March 1951, Ms. ZHU published her monograph *Xin Zhenjiu Xue* (《新针灸学》*The New Acupuncture and Moxibustion*) which was the first major book for "exploring improvement of techniques and scientific mechanisms of acupuncture-moxibustion by applying modern scientific theory and methodology". Later on, her book was translated into and published in multilingual versions, such as Korean, Russian, Vietnamese, etc. After the founding of the People's Republic of China, Ms. ZHU founded the Experimental Institute of Acupuncture and Moxibustion Therapeutics (current Institute of Acupuncture and Moxibustion, CACMS), directly subordinated to the Health Ministry of People's Central Government and was appointed head of the institution.

"Slowly-twirling inserting method of acupuncture needle" concluded by Ms. Zhu, also known as "ZHU Lian's Needling Technique", has become one of the needling methods of "Guangxi Acupuncture School", and her invented "moxa-roll-hanging moxibustion" and "needle-embedding" techniques have been being frequently applied in clinic practice nowadays.

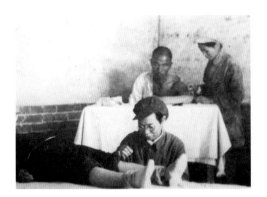

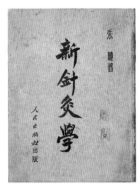

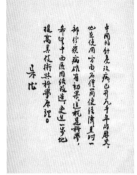

◇朱琏用针灸治病（1946 年 4 月）

抗战期间，朱琏在太行山革命根据地开展针灸治疗工作

Ms. ZHU Lian using acupuncture needle to treat a patient (Taken in April 1946)
Ms. ZHU Lian treated patients with acupuncture and moxibustion in the Taihang Mountain revolutionary base during the Anti-Japanese War

◇《新针灸学》封面及朱德题词

人民卫生出版社，1951 年第 1 版

The cover page of *Xin Zhenjiu Xue* and ZHU De's epigraph
The 1st edition of *Xin Zhenjiu Xue*, published by the People's Medical Publishing House

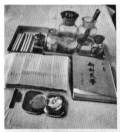

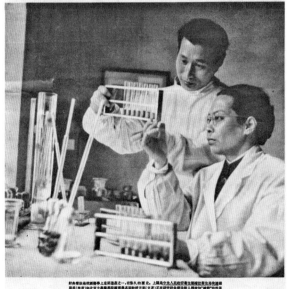

◇朱琏在研究针灸疗法对人体增加"补体"效果

引自《人民画报》，1952 年 1 月

ZHU Lian studying the "reinforcing effect" of acupuncture-moxibustion therapies on human body
Cited from *China Pictorial* in January 1952

## 艾卷灸的来历

1951 年夏天，朱琏去上海开会，在列车上突发急性肠炎。她想用灸法自治，却又没带艾绒，于是她从兜里掏出一盒香烟，抽出一根点燃，然后对准大肠俞、足三里等穴悬起熏烤，病症得到很好的缓解，香烟卷熏灸起到了与艾炷灸相似的疗效。朱琏觉得很有意思，此后经她反复试验，发现这种熏灸法不仅疗效确切，还可随时调整所需热力大小，减少了施灸中的许多麻烦。于是，朱琏指示她所领导的卫生部针灸疗法实验所开展研究，分别运用艾卷灸和艾炷灸在"合谷"穴上施灸，观察其皮肤温度的变化，结果表明艾卷灸法不但使用方便，而且在温度的调节上也比艾炷灸法优越。之后，针灸疗法实验所将"艾卷灸"用于临床治病，并将此疗法陆续推广至全国，这就是后来大家所熟知的"艾条悬起灸法"的来历。

## The origin of moxibustion with moxa-stick

In the summer of 1951, on her way to Shanghai for a meeting, ZHU Lian had an attack of acute enteritis on the train. She would like to use moxibustion to treat herself, but she did not bring any moxa with her at that moment. So she took out a box of cigarettes from her pocket and ignited one of them. Then she applied moxibustion over the points of Dachangshu (BL 25), Zusanli (ST 36), etc. with the ignited cigarette, and her symptoms were alleviated soon. Her personal experience suggested that moxibustion with cigarettes had similar functions as those of moxibustion with moxa cones.

ZHU Lian thought that it was very interesting. After repeated experiments, she found that such kind of moxibustion not only had a definite effect, but also could adjust the required heat at any time, and avoid a lot of troubles during moxibustion. So she proposed to carry out the research on moxibustion in the Experimental Institute of Acupuncture and Moxibustion Therapeutics subordinating to the Ministry of Health under her leadership.

During the research, moxa sticks and moxa cones were applied successively at the point Hegu (LI 4) for observation of the changes of skin temperature. The result showed that moxibustion with moxa sticks was not only convenient for application, but also superior in adjusting warmth to that of moxa cones. After the research, the Experimental Institute of Acupuncture and Moxibustion Therapeutics decided to put "moxibustion with moxa sticks" into clinical practice and make the therapy popular step by step in the whole country. This is the story about "hanging moxibustion with moxa sticks".

# 65

## 中央人民政府卫生部针灸疗法实验所
### Experimental Institute of Acupuncture and Moxibustion Therapeutics subordinating to the Health Ministry of People's Central Government

1951年8月,中央人民政府卫生部针灸疗法实验所在朱琏等人倡导和努力下创立,成为我国第一家针灸研究机构,主要开展针灸医疗、教学、实验、对外交流等工作,初创及发展过程中得到毛泽东、周恩来、朱德、董必武等老一辈革命家的关心、爱护与支持。1955年12月,中医研究院成立,中央人民政府卫生部针灸疗法实验所更名为中医研究院针灸研究所,成为国内最大的针灸科研机构,也是世界卫生组织传统医学(针灸)合作中心。

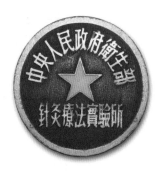

◇针灸疗法实验所纪念胸章

Commemorative badge of the EIAMT

In August of 1951, Ms. ZHU Lian founded the Experimental Institute of Acupuncture and Moxibustion Therapeutics (EIAMT) directly subordinating to Health Ministry of People's Central Government, the first acupuncture-moxibustion research institution in China. This institute mainly focused on clinical treatment, education, animal experiments, and foreign exchanges. During its founding and development, many older generation of revolutionaries and senior leaders of the People's Central Government of China, such as Chairman MAO Ze-dong, Prime Minister ZHOU En-lai, ZHU De (the Chairman of the Standing Committee of the People's Congress), Vice President

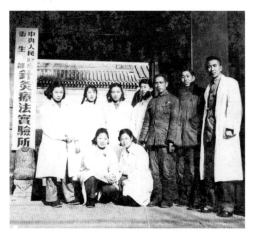

◇针灸疗法实验所部分工作人员留影(1953年冬)

A group photo of some staffs of the EIAMT
Taken in the winter of 1953

DONG Bi-wu, et al gave a lot of care, cherishing and supports. In December 1955, China Academy of Traditional Chinese medicine was set up. The EIAMT was renamed as the Institute of Acupuncture and Moxibustion of China Academy of Traditional Chinese medicine. The institute is now the largest institution for acupuncture research in China, and WHO Collaborating Centre for Traditional Medicine (Acupuncture).

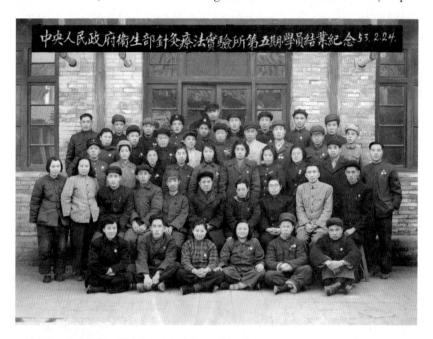

◇针灸疗法实验所第五期学员结业纪念（1953年2月）

Graduation memorial picture of students of the 5<sup>th</sup> session of the EIAMT
Taken in February of 1953

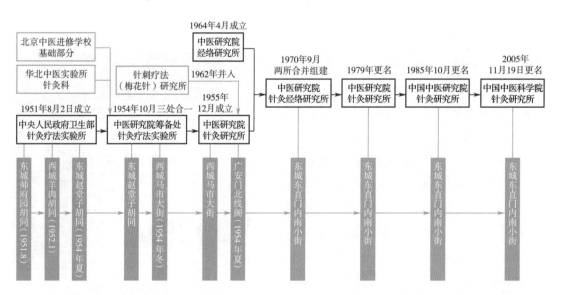

◇从针灸疗法实验所到针灸研究所历史变迁

Historical changes from the EIAMT to the Institute of Acupuncture and Moxibustion

# 66

## 毛泽东主席说"针灸不是土东西"

## Chairman MAO Ze-dong said that "acupuncture and moxibustion are not unscientific things"

1955 年 4 月 15 日,毛泽东主席在杭州接见卫生部针灸疗法实验所所长朱琏,毛主席颇为赞同朱琏《新针灸学》一书中关于针灸与现代医学理论发展的关系问题,晚餐席间举杯"祝针灸万岁",并指出"针灸不是土东西,针灸是科学的,将来世界各国都要用它"。毛主席还曾指示:针灸是中医里面的精华之精华,要好好地推广、研究,它将来发展前途很广。

On April 15th, 1955 at Hangzhou, Chairman MAO Ze-dong met with Ms. ZHU Lian (the head of the EIAMT of the Ministry of Health) and expressed his approval of ZHU's viewpoints about the theoretical development of acupuncture-moxibustion and modern medicine in ZHU's book *Xin Zhenjiu Xue*. During supper, Chairman MAO even proposed a toast to "long live acupuncture and moxibustion" at dinner table, and pointed out that "acupuncture and moxibustion are not unscientific things, but rather scientific, and will be employed worldwide." Chairman MAO even once emphasized that acupuncture and moxibustion are the most essential component of TCM and have a wonderful prospect in the future, and thus should be well popularized and well studied.

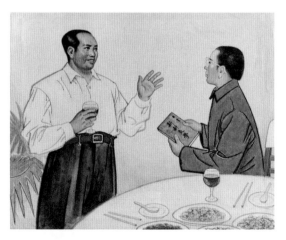

◇毛泽东主席在杭州接见朱琏画
**摄于河北省双凤山革命陵园朱琏生平展室**

Chairman MAO meeting with ZHU Lian in Hangzhou
Photographed at the exhibition-hall of ZHU Lian, in the cemetery for revolutionists, at Shuangfengshan, Hebei Province

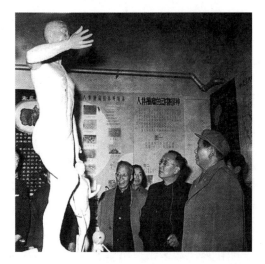

◇毛泽东主席观看人体经络穴位模型

1958 年 10 月 27 日,毛泽东主席由郭沫若(右 2)陪同,参观了中国科学院自然科学展览会,图片引自《北京卫生志》

Chairman MAO Ze-dong, was carefully looking at the human model with meridians and acupoints
On October 27th, 1958, Chairman MAO Ze-dong, visited the Natural Science Exhibition of China Academy of Science, accompanied by Mr. GUO Mo-ruo (the second one from the right), quoted from *Beijing Weisheng Zhi* (《北京卫生志》*Beijing's Health Chronicles*)

##  毛泽东主席在广州接见朱琏

1958 年 4 月 19 日,毛泽东主席在广州接见朱琏,也成为针灸发展史上的重要事件。见面后毛主席第一句话就问:"办了针灸学院吗？"早在 1951 年成立针灸疗法实验所时,朱琏就曾设想建立"针灸实验院",建立大规模的针灸研究院,附设针灸学院和医院,事隔多年,毛主席关心针灸研究的发展,心中一直记挂此事。会谈中毛主席特别询问了中医研究院中医研究班的情况,还发表了对中西医的看法:"我看西医治感冒就很少有办法,中医治感冒有时一副药就治好了。替我治感冒的中医就是用一副药。"之后,主席详细询问了苏联派遣 3 位医学专家学习针灸及她们回国后开展工作的情况,指示苏联办全苏性的针灸训练班,我们也要给予帮助。主席还询问了针灸治疗疟疾、痢疾、血吸虫病的工作,及针灸在各省市开办训练班的情况,朱琏均给予认真汇报。主席还非常关心针灸治疗癌瘤的情况,朱琏举两例说明在农村用针灸治疗肿瘤,听后,主席兴奋地连声说:"有名堂,有名堂,针灸也许可以治疗癌病！"

此次接见后,1958 年 10 月,毛主席在对卫生部党组 9 月 25 日关于西医学中医离职学习班的总结报告上作了重要批示,指出"中国医药学是一个伟大的宝库,应当努力发掘,加以提高。"之后西医学习中医迅速掀起了一个新的高潮,多种形式的"西学中"教育培养了一大批中西医兼通的新型人才。

## Chairman MAO Ze-dong met ZHU Lian in Guangzhou

On April 19, 1958, Chairman MAO Ze-dong met ZHU Lian in Guangzhou, which became an important event in the history of acupuncture and moxibustion. As soon as they met, Chairman MAO asked: "Has the College of Acupuncture and Moxibustion been set up?" As early as 1951 when the Experimental Institute of Acupuncture and Moxibustion Therapeutics was founded, ZHU Lian had envisaged the establishment of "An Acupuncture and Moxibustion Academy", a large-scale Acupuncture and Moxibustion Research Institute, with colleges and hospitals attached. After many years, Chairman MAO was concerned about the development of acupuncture and moxibustion research. During the talks, Chairman MAO inquired about the research course of TCM in the Academy of Traditional Chinese Medicine, and expressed his views on Chinese and Western medicine: "I think there are few ways to treat a cold in Western medicine, but sometimes a dose of Chinese herbal medicine can treat a cold. The doctor once cured me when I caught a cold only by prescribing one dose of Chinese herbal medicine". After that, the Chairman inquired in detail about the three medical experts sent by the Soviet Union to study acupuncture and their work after going back home. He pointed out that an acupuncture and moxibustion training course could be run nationwide in the Soviet Union, and we should support them. Chairman MAO also asked about treatment of malaria, dysentery and schistosomiasis with acupuncture and moxibustion, and the training courses of acupuncture and moxibustion in various provinces and cities. ZHU Lian answered and reported in detail. Chairman MAO was also very concerned about acupuncture and moxibustion therapies in the treatment of cancer. ZHU Lian gave two examples of treatment of cancer in the countryside with acupuncture and moxibustion. After listening, Chairman MAO said excitedly, "Great! It's possible and hopeful that cancer may be treated by acupuncture and moxibustion."

Following this interview, in October 1958, Chairman MAO made an important instruction in the summary report of the Party group of the Ministry of Health on September 25th on a full-time training course for doctors of Western medicine learning Chinese medicine. He pointed out that "Chinese medicine is a great treasure house, which should be explored and improved with great efforts". After that, doctors of Western medicine learning Chinese medicine reached a new climax and a large number of new talents with knowledge of both Chinese and Western medicine were trained in various forms of education.

# 67

# 首批来华学习针灸的外国专家小组
The first foreign expert group to study acupuncture and moxibustion in China

1956 年 4 月 14 日—7 月 14 日，根据中苏技术交流协定，苏联保健部派国家保健机构及医学史研究所的德柯琴斯卡亚教授、莫斯科中央医师进修学院的神经科医师乌索娃、神经理疗科医师奥辛波娃 3 人来华组成专家小组，到中国中医研究院针灸研究所考察学习针灸疗法，了解包括中国各种门诊和医院治疗机构使用针灸方法的情况、针灸使用技术和方法方面的理论与实际的研究等专题。这是第一个来华考察学习针灸疗法的外国专家小组，被列入《建国以来医药卫生大事记》。当时，针灸研究所选派学术造诣很深的针灸专家为 3 位医师专门举办针灸学习班，传授系统的针灸学知识。她们学成回国后，开展针灸临床和科研工作，成为针灸骨干，推动了针灸学在苏联的传播。

From April 14<sup>th</sup> to July 14<sup>th</sup>, 1956, according to a technical exchange agreement between Chinese and Soviet Union governments, a delegation consisting of 3 experts, Prof. Dekchinskaya (from the Soviet Health Care Institution and the Medical History Institute), Usova (a neurologist of Moscow Central Physician Training College) and Osinpova (a neuro-physiotherapist of the Neurophysiotherapy Department of the Moscow Central Physician Training College) was sent to China to investigate and study acupuncture and moxibustion therapies in the Institute of Acupuncture and Moxibustion of China Academy of Traditional Chinese Medicine (current CACMS) by the Soviet Ministry of Health. They also wanted to investigate the state of application of acupuncture-moxibustion in various outpatient departments and hospitals, and researches on the theory and clinical practice of acupuncture-moxibustion techniques. That was the first foreign specialist group visiting China for studying these therapies, which has been included in *Jianguoyilai Yiyaoweisheng Dashiji* (《建国以来医药卫生大事记》*The Medical and Health Memorabilia since the Founding of the People's Republic of China*). At that time, the Institute of Acupuncture and Moxibustion chose 3 highly-qualified acupuncturists to open a special training class for them. After returning to their home country, the 3 Soviet experts conducted acupuncture clinical treatment and scientific research, and became the backbones in this field, pushing forward the popularization of acupuncture and moxibustion in Soviet Union.

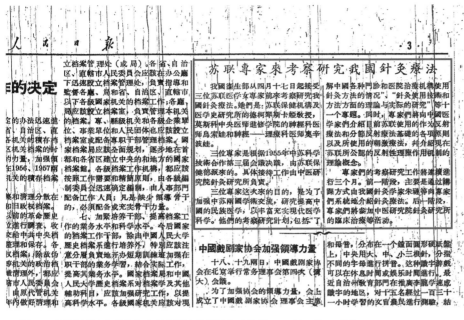

◇《人民日报》报道"苏联专家来考察研究我国针灸疗法"（1956 年 4 月 21 日）

A report of *People's Daily* titled "Soviet experts visited our country to investigate and study Chinese acupuncture and moxibustion therapies" (April 21st, 1956)

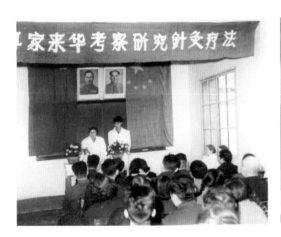

◇针灸研究所召开欢迎会

Welcome ceremony held in the Institute of Acupuncture and Moxibustion

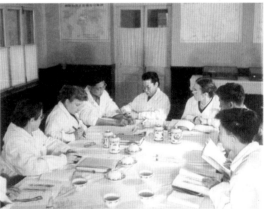

◇针灸研究所专家指导苏联专家理论学习

Chinese expert giving a lecture on TCM theories to the Soviet experts

◇针灸研究所欢送苏联专家回国合影（1956 年 7 月 16 日）欢送会

A group photo of 3 Soviet experts and Chinese experts and leaders from the Institute of Acupuncture and Moxibustion before a farewell meeting (July 16th, 1956)

# 68

# 现代毫针的发展
## Development of modern filiform needle

毫针是针灸临床上最常用的针具。20世纪40年代以前,毫针材质多以铁为主,也有用金、银制造的,并且多为手工制作,这一时期的毫针一般较粗。至1953年,在承澹盦先生的倡导下,开始制造不锈钢质的毫针,并逐渐规范其规格,毫针质量的提高大大推动了针灸的推广和发展。此后,针灸疗法开始逐步走向世界,为适应新的要求,出现了目前为临床广泛使用的一次性无菌毫针。

The filiform needle is the most commonly-used acupuncture needle in clinic. Before 1940s, the filiform needle was mainly made of iron, and sometimes also made of gold or silver, and mostly being handmade. At that time, the filiform needle was often thicker. In 1953, under the advocacy of Mr. CHENG Dan-an, the stainless steel began to be utilized and the specifications were standardized gradually. The improvement of the quality of the filiform needle greatly gives impetus to the popularization and development of acupuncture therapy. Thereafter, acupuncture therapy began to go to the world step by step. Moreover, a disposable sterile filiform needle becomes popular in clinical practice for adapting patients' new requirements.

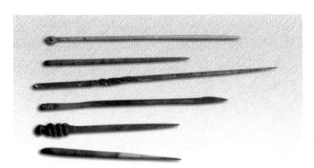

◇民国针具
　张赞臣捐赠,河南南阳医圣祠所藏

Acupuncture needles used during the Republic of China
Donated by Mr. ZHANG Zan-chen, preserved in the Temple of Medical Saint at Nanyang of Henan Province

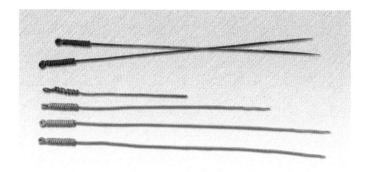

◇ 20 世纪 40 年代金银针

朱琏在延安、太行山区使用过，中国中医科学院针灸研究所针灸博物馆藏

Gold and silver acupuncture needles available in 1940s
Acupuncture needles used by Ms. ZHU Lian in Yan'an and Taihang Mountain region, collected by the Chinese Museum of Acupuncture and Moxibustion, Institute of Acupuncture and Moxibustion, CACMS

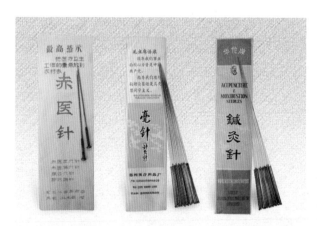

◇ 20 世纪 70 年代毫针

Filiform needles made in 1970s

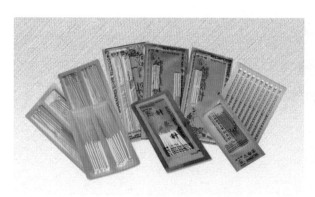

◇各种毫针

苏州医疗用品厂有限公司制造

New types of filiform needles
Made by Suzhou Medical Appliance Factory Co. Ltd.

**一次性无菌毫针**

一次性无菌毫针,是经过特殊方法灭菌的毫针,通常使用环氧乙烷灭菌法,使用时不需再行灭菌消毒,即拆即用,用后即弃。一次性无菌毫针的推广和使用受到了广大患者的欢迎,促进了传统针灸的国际传播。世界针灸学会联合会前主席陈绍武教授曾说过,如果没有一次性毫针行销世界,各国政府承认针灸医学的合法性就不会那么容易。

## Disposable sterile needles

Disposable sterile filiform needles are made by a special method of sterilization with ethyleneoxide. For usage, just open the package and take the needle out. They are convenient to use and disposable after being used. The popularization and use of disposable aseptic filiform needles have been well accepted by patients and promoted the international spread of traditional acupuncture and moxibustion. Prof. CHEN Shao-wu, former chairman of the World Federation of Acupuncture and Moxibustion Societies, once said that it would not be easy for governments of the foreign countries to acknowledge the legality of acupuncture and moxibustion medicine without worldwide sale of disposable needles.

# 69

# 高等教育针灸学教材
## Teaching materials for acupuncture-moxibustion in Chinese higher education

高等教育针灸学统编教材,分中医专业和针灸专业两类。

中医专业的针灸教材,第 1 版是 1961 年由南京中医学院(现南京中医药大学)针灸教研组编著、人民卫生出版社出版的中医学院试用教材《针灸学讲义》(其前身是 1957 年 10 月该教研组编著、江苏人民出版社出版的《针灸学》),1964 年重新修订后再版,1972 年该版第 3 次印刷时更名为《针灸学》。

20 世纪 80 年代编第 5 版中医专业教材《针灸学》时,为适应针灸学科发展的需要,开始编撰专供针灸专业使用的教材,包括《经络学》《腧穴学》《刺法灸法学》《针灸治疗学》《针灸医籍选》《各家针灸学说》。

The state-compiled textbook on acupuncture and moxibustion for higher education is classified into two categories: TCM speciality and acupuncture-moxibustion speciality.

In October 1957, *Zhenjiu Xue* (《针灸学》*Acupuncture and Moxibustion*) was complied by the Teaching and Research Section of Acupuncture-Moxibustion of Nanjing College of TCM (current Nanjing University of CM) and published by Jiangsu People's Publishing House. This book is the predecessor of *Zhenjiuxue Jiangyi* (《针灸学讲义》*Teaching Material of Acupuncture and Moxibustion*), a teaching material on probation for colleges of TCM in China (in 1961) compiled by Nanjing College of TCM, published by the People's Medical Publishing House. That is the first edition of textbook *Acupuncture and Moxibustion*, the uniformly-compiled teaching material for TCM subject of higher education in China. In 1964, it was revised and reprinted once again. In 1972, it was still named as *Zhenjiu Xue* when reprinted for the $3^{rd}$ time.

When compiling the $5^{th}$ edition textbook of *Zhenjiu Xue* for TCM specialty of colleges and universities of TCM in 1980s, a set of uniformly-complied textbooks exclusively used for acupuncture-moxibustion speciality began to be written, including *Jingluo Xue* (《经络学》*Meridian-collateral Learnings*), *Shuxue Xue* (《腧穴学》*Acupoints Learnings*), *Cifa Jiufa Xue* (《刺法灸法学》*Acupuncture-moxibustion*

*Techniques), Zhenjiu Zhiliao Xue (《针灸治疗学》Therapeutics of Acupuncture and Moxibustion), Zhenjiu Yiji Xuan (《针灸医籍选》Collection of the Selected Medical Classic on Acupuncture and Moxibustion), Gejia Zhenjiu Xueshuo (《各家针灸学说》Various Schools of Acupuncture and Moxibustion), etc. to meet the requirements of spreading acupuncture and moxibustion.*

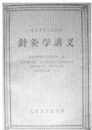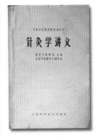

◇第1版、2版中医学院试用教材《针灸学讲义》
南京中医学院针灸教研组编，人民卫生出版社，1961年

*Zhenjiuxue Jiangyi*, the 1st and 2nd editions of trial teaching materials for TCM colleges
Compiled by the Teaching-research Section of Acupuncture-moxibustion of Nanjing College of TCM, published by the People's Medical Publishing House in 1961

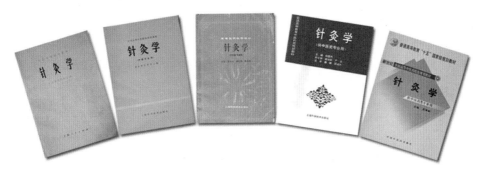

◇第3~7版《针灸学》

The 3rd to 7th editions of textbook *Zhenjiu Xue*

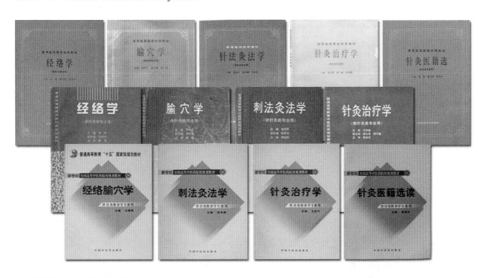

◇各版针灸专业针灸统编教材

Different editions of the state-compiled textbooks of acupuncture-moxibustion speciality

### 第一部针灸对外培训教材

20世纪50年代，随着国际文化交流的日益加强，不少友好国家先后选派医师来我国考察和研究针灸疗法，产生了很大兴趣，希望能更多地了解针灸学知识。1959年，卫生部召集北京中医学院（现北京中医药大学）、上海中医学院（现上海中医药大学）、南京中医学院（现南京中医药大学）和中医研究院（现中国中医科学院）针灸研究所的针灸专家，联合编写我国第一部针灸对外培训教材——《中国针灸学概要》，于1964年6月由人民卫生出版社出版，作为国外医师学习针灸的培训教材。1977年译成法文第1版，由外文出版社（北京）出版。1979年，该书中文版修订再版，并于1980年译成英文第1版，由外文出版社出版。1986年7月，经修订增补更名为《中国针灸学》出版，作为中国中医研究院、上海中医学院、南京中医学院三家国际针灸培训班的教材。该书的出版对针灸学的国际传播起到了积极的推进作用，在针灸对外教学中影响很大。

## The first textbook of acupuncture and moxibustion for international training

In the 1950s, along with the increasing international cultural exchanges, many friendly countries sent doctors to China to study acupuncture and moxibustion therapies. They were very interested in TCM, hoping to know more about acupuncture and moxibustion. In 1959, the Ministry of Health convened acupuncturists from Beijing College of TCM (current Beijing University of CM), Shanghai College of TCM (current Shanghai University of TCM), Nanjing College of TCM (current Nanjing University of CM) and the Institute of Acupuncture and Moxibustion of China Academy of Traditional Chinese Medicine, Beijing to compile the first textbook on acupuncture and moxibustion for international training, *Zhongguo Zhenjiu Xue Gaiyao* (《中国针灸学概要》*Essentials of Chinese Acupuncture*) which was published by the People's Medical Publishing House in June 1964 as a training material for foreign doctors to study Chinese acupuncture and moxibustion. In 1977, the book was translated into French, and the first edition was published by the Foreign Language Press (Beijing). In 1979, the Chinese version of the book was revised and republished, and in 1980 it was translated into English and the first edition was published by the Foreign Language Publishing House. In July 1986, the book was revised again and renamed as *Zhongguo Zhenjiu Xue* as the textbook for foreign students in three international acupuncture training centers, the Institute of Acupuncture and Moxibustion, China Academy of Traditional Chinese Medicine, Shanghai College of TCM and Nanjing College of TCM respectively.

The publication of the book has played a positive role in promoting the international dissemination of acupuncture and moxibustion, and has a great impact on the international education of acupuncture and moxibustion.

# 70

## 针灸传入非洲
## Introduction of acupuncture to Africa

20 世纪 60 年代初，中国政府派遣援非医疗队，开启了针灸传入非洲的大门，如 1965 年 10 月中医研究院派出针灸医生参加中国援非医疗队，在非洲开展中国针灸疗法。此后，中国政府每年都派遣医疗队分赴非洲各国，共向约 50 个非洲国家派出 2 万余人次的医疗队员，使 2 亿多非洲人民得到无偿医疗援助。援非医疗队中的针灸医生，是在非洲从事针灸工作的主体，用针灸治疗艾滋病并发症、腰腿痛、疟疾、消瘦、变态反应性疾病等几十种疾病。除临床诊疗外，援非医疗队的针灸医生们还在当地培养了一批医务人员，为针灸在非洲的传播与发展打下了基础。

除援非医疗队外，自 20 世纪 70 年代起，我国还开展了不同层次的对外中医教育。据统计，从非洲来华学习中医者已逾千人，几乎遍布非洲的所有国家和地区。

At the beginning of 1960s, Chinese government sent medical aid teams to Africa, opening a door to the introduction of acupuncture-moxibustion to Africa. In October 1965, China Academy of Traditional Chinese medicine sent acupuncturists to joint Chinese medical aid team to Africa to serve the local people by using acupuncture and moxibustion therapies. Since then, Chinese government has been yearly sending medical aid teams to many countries of Africa. Up to now, more than 20,000 Chinese medical staff offered free medical aid to over 200 million people of about 50 African countries. Chinese acupuncturists are the main members of all the experts working in Africa. They employed acupuncture and moxibustion therapies to treat dozens of problems, such as complications of AIDS, lumbago, leg pain, malaria, emaciation, allergic diseases, etc. Chinese doctors not only devoted themselves to medical practice there, but also cultivated many local medical staff, laying the foundation for the dissemination and development of acupuncture-moxibustion in Africa. Since 1970s, China has also carried out education of different levels of TCM apart from sending medical aid teams to Africa. Statistically, more than 1,000 practitioners from almost every country or region of Africa have studied TCM in China.

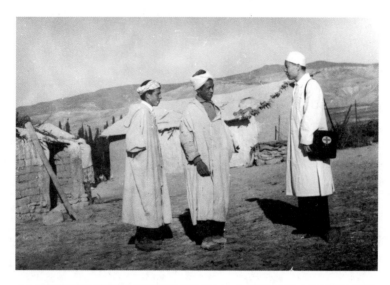

◇中医研究院针灸研究所援非医疗队田从豁（右1）在阿尔及利亚萨哈拉牧区巡诊
（1966年）

Prof. TIAN Cong-huo (the first from the right), a member of the medical aid team to Africa from the Institute of Acupuncture and Moxibustion, China Academy of TCM, was offering a round of medical visits to Sahara pastoral area, Algeria in 1966

# 71

# 重复朝鲜凤汉系统实验
## Experiments for reproducing North Korean "Bonghan System"

1963 年 11 月,朝鲜金凤汉教授在朝鲜医学期刊发表报告,宣布发现了与中国古代经脉经穴相对应的解剖结构,命名为凤汉系统,获当年度"金日成"奖,这引起中国政府的重视。为重复金凤汉的工作,我国 2 次组织相关领域的一流专家赴朝鲜学习考察。1964 年 4 月,在中医研究院组建"经络研究所",由全国 10 家医学研究机构的专家组成专业科研队伍专门研究凤汉系统。在获得大量实验数据的基础上,证伪了凤汉系统理论。此项工作,为我国日后经络实质的研究奠定了一定的基础,为针灸的现代研究培养了一批重要的科研人才。

In November 1963, Prof. Bonghan KIM from the Democratic People's Republic of Korea (DPRK) declared on the *Journal of the DPRK Academy of Medical Science* that he found the anatomical structure of classical meridians and meridian acupoints and named them Bonghan corpuscles (BHCs) and Bonghan ducts (BHDs) system. Hence, he was awarded with "Kim Il-sung" prize in the same year. This event drew great attention from Chinese government. In order to confirm KIM's results, China organized first-class experts of the related fields to visit DPRK twice. In April 1964, the Institute of Meridian-collaterals was established under China Academy of TCM in Beijing. Experts from more than 10 medical colleges and research institutes of China began to devote themselves to reproduce the "Bonghan system". Following a series of experiments, Chinese researchers obtained a large amount of experimental data, and disproved the so-called "Bonghan system" at last. In spite of this, this work built on a certain foundation for China's future research on the essence of meridian-collaterals, and cultivated a number of important scientific research personnels for the modern study of acupuncture-moxibustion.

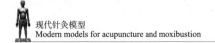

# 72

## 现代针灸模型
## Modern models for acupuncture and moxibustion

在古代,政府就非常重视针灸模型的铸造,如宋元明清时期铸有多具针灸铜人。20世纪50年代以后,运用现代声、光、电技术,陆续研制出了多种材质的针灸经穴人体模型,如针灸经穴玻璃人模型等,通入电流时能生动清晰地显示经穴位置、经络循行及其与脏腑的关系。1987年10月,国家组织专家多方考证,重铸宋天圣针灸铜人成功,于2007年列入第一批河南省省级非物质文化遗产名录。

目前最常用的针灸模型是塑料材质的,它按人体大小等比缩小,便于携带学习。

In ancient China, the central government thought highly of casting acupuncture figures. For example, in the Song, Yuan, Ming and Qing Dynasties, many bronze acupuncture figures were cast. After 1950s, acupuncture and meridian-acupoint models made from multiple types of materials were developed successively by using modern sound, light and electric techniques. For instance, the acupuncture meridian-acupoint glass manikin model which is able to clearly display the acupoint location, and the interrelation between the meridian running course and the related internal organs was developed. In October 1987, Chinese government convened experts to conduct systematic research and successfully recast the Tiansheng Acupuncture Bronze Figure of the Song Dynasty which was inscribed on the first batch of list of provincial-class intangible cultural heritage by the government of Henan Province in 2007.

At the present, the most commonly-used acupuncture model is made up of plastic material, and is miniaturized in the light of the size of human body for the convenience of carrying and study.

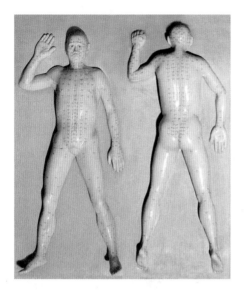

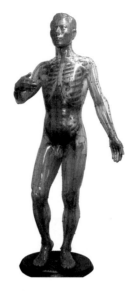

◇人体经穴模型

　人高60cm，1954年赵尔康先生设计，中国中医科学院针灸研究所针灸博物馆藏

Human model with acupoints (60cm in height)
Designed by Mr. ZHAO Er-kang in 1954, collected by the Chinese Museum of Acupuncture and Moxibustion of the Institute of Acupuncture and Moxibustion, CACMS

◇针灸经穴玻璃人模型

　人高160cm，中国中医科学院针灸研究所针灸博物馆藏（1963年）

Glass-manikin with meridian-acupuncture points (160cm in height)
Collected by the Chinese Museum of Acupuncture and Moxibustion of the Institute of Acupuncture and Moxibustion, CACMS (1963)

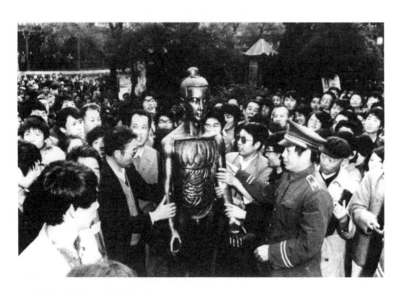

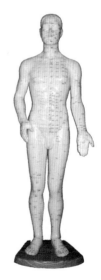

◇开封市重铸宋天圣针灸铜人

　河南省开封市大相国寺收藏（1987年）

Recast Tiansheng Acupuncture Bronze Figure of the Song Dynasty in Kaifeng City
Collected by Daxiangguo Temple in Kaifeng City, Henan Province (1987)

◇针灸经穴塑料人模型

　人高50cm，苏州医疗用品厂有限公司制造

Plastic manikin of acupuncture points (50cm in height)
Made by Suzhou Medical Appliance Factory Co. Ltd.

# 73

## 电针仪的发展
## Development of electroacupuncture apparatus

1825 年法国萨朗弟爱（Sarlandière）出版了电针著作，从而使他成为电针疗法的创始人。1930 年，日本在临床上开始使用电针。1933 年，唐世丞等人将电子管产生的脉冲电流应用于临床，研制出我国第 1 批电针仪。1953 年，朱龙玉开始在临床上推广使用电针仪。自 1958 年始，电针仪用于针刺麻醉取得成功。之后，电针仪在针灸临床、科研领域发挥了重要作用。20 世纪 80 年代末，辛育龄研制出电化学癌症治疗仪，以针形电极作为针具刺入瘤体治疗癌症。1991 年，韩济生和刘亦鸣共同研制了"韩氏穴位神经刺激仪"，对镇痛和治疗海洛因成瘾具有良好疗效。2007 年，朱兵和曹炀研制出一种由针刺手法刺激引发的生物信息针疗仪，适合临床针灸个体化治疗及科研量化。

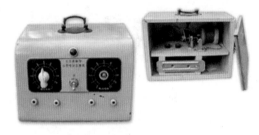

◇ 20 世纪 50 年代针灸治疗仪

采用机械方式产生脉冲刺激信号，中国中医科学院针灸研究所针灸博物馆藏

The EA apparatus made in 1950s, being able to produce pulse stimulus signals via mechanical way, collected by Chinese Museum of Acupuncture and Moxibustion of the Institute of Acupuncture and Moxibustion, CACMS

In 1825, French Jean-Baptiste Sarlandière published his book *Electroacupuncture* that made him the father of electroacupuncture (EA) therapy. Japanese began to apply EA clinically in 1930. Chinese TANG Shi-cheng and his colleagues invented the first batch of EA apparatuses and applied pulse current produced

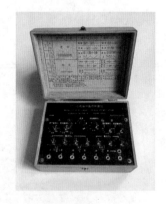

◇ 57-6 型电脉冲医疗刺激仪

20 世纪 70—80 年代使用较多的针灸电针仪，北京航空学院（现北京航空航天大学）制

57-6 Type Medical Electro-pulse Therapeutic Stimulator (employed more frequently from 1970s to 1980s) Developed by Beijing Aeronautics College (current Beihang University)

from electron tubes to clinical practice. In 1953, ZHU Yu-long took the lead in popularizing EA apparatus in clinic. Since 1958, EA apparatus has been successfully applied to acupuncture anesthesia. Afterwards, the EA apparatus plays an important role in acupuncture clinic and scientific research.

At the end of 1980s, Prof. XIN Yu-ling invented an Electrochemical Therapeutic Apparatus for cancers on the body surface by inserting needle-shaped electrodes into the tumor mass. In 1991, Prof. HAN Ji-sheng and LIU Yi-ming jointly developed Han's Acupoint Nerve Stimulator (HANS) which has a good therapeutic effect in relieving pain and Heroin addiction. In 2007, Prof. ZHU Bin and CAO Yang invented Bioinformatic Acupuncture Manipulation Therapeutic Apparatus which can simulate manual needle stimulation, being applicable for individualized treatment and scientific research quantization.

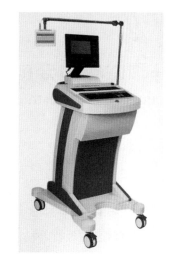

◇育龄牌 ZAY-6B 型电化学治疗仪
引自第八届电化学治疗肿瘤国际会议论文集（2004 年 9 月）

Yuling Brand ZAY-6B Electrochemical Therapeutic Apparatus
Cited from the paper collection of The 8th International Symposium on Electrochemical Therapy for Tumor (September 2004)

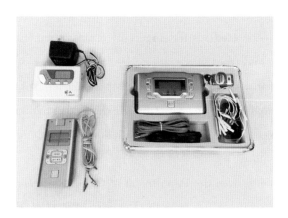

◇韩氏穴位神经刺激仪

Han's Acupoint Nerve Stimulator

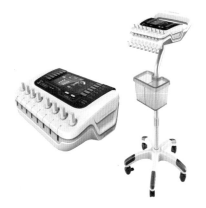

◇ SXDZ-200（Ⅲ代）针刺手法针疗仪

SXDZ-200（Ⅲ）Bioinformatic Acupuncture Manipulation Therapeutic Apparatus

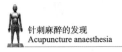
# 74

## 针刺麻醉的发现
Acupuncture anaesthesia

　　针刺麻醉（简称针麻）是根据手术部位、手术病种等，选穴针刺以获得麻醉效果，在患者处于清醒状态时施行外科手术的一种麻醉方法，是古老针刺止痛与现代外科手术相结合的产物。针刺麻醉的发现，是我国传统的针灸医学在现代的一次重大突破，是 20 世纪针灸学科中最重要的原创性成果之一。

　　1958 年 8 月 30 日，上海市第一人民医院耳鼻喉科尹惠珠医生和该院中医科合作，第一次以针刺代替药物麻醉，成功实施第一例针麻手术——扁桃体摘除术，创造了突破性的记录；1958 年 12 月 5 日，西安市第四人民医院首次运用电针开展针刺麻醉。1971 年 7 月 19 日，我国新华社以"我国医务工作者和科学工作者创造成功针刺麻醉"为题，首次向全世界正式宣布了这一消息，引起国内外医学界的强烈反响和关注。

Acupuncture anesthesia is one of the analgesic methods for surgery by means of puncturing the selected acupoints according to the location and types of operation when the patient is still in conscious state. It is a conjunctive product of the ancient acupuncture analgesia and modern surgery. The discovery of acupuncture anesthesia is a breakthrough of modern China in the field of traditional acupuncture-moxibustion medicine, and is one of the most important original achievements in acupuncture-moxibustion dicipline in the 20th century.

On August 30th, 1958, YIN Hui-zhu, a doctor from the Department of Otorhinolaryngology of Shanghai First People's Hospital, co-operated with doctors from the Department of TCM of the same hospital to successfully conduct tonsillectomy, the 1st case of surgical operation by using acupuncture anesthesia, creating a breakthrough recording in China. On December 5th, 1958, the 4th People's Hospital of Xi'an City applied electro-acupuncture anesthesia to clinic for the first time. On July 19th, 1971, Chinese Xinhua News Agency formally announced the news titled "Chinese medical workers and scientists successfully create acupuncture anesthesia" to the world, causing stronger responses and attention in the medical community both at home and abroad.

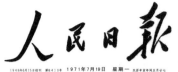

**毛主席语录**

在生产斗争和科学实验范围内，人类总是不断发展的，自然界也总是不断发展的，永远不会停止在一个水平上。

1948年6月15日创刊 第8410号　1971年7月19日　星期一

## 毛主席无产阶级卫生路线和科研路线的伟大胜利

# 我国医务工作者和科学工作者创造成功针刺麻醉

### 周恩来总理郭沫若副委员长
### 会见法国议会代表团

## 中西医结合的光辉范例

—— 欢呼我国创造成功针刺麻醉

（一）

（二）

（三）

（下转第三版）

◇ 1971 年新华社首次向全世界正式
公布针麻成果

The first authorized announcement on the
success of acupuncture anaesthesia was
made formally by Chinese Xinhua News
Agency in 1971

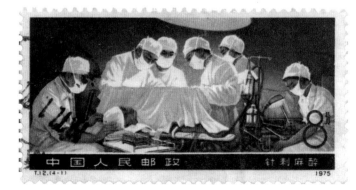

◇针刺麻醉邮票

1976 年 4 月 9 日发行，周建杨教授藏

A stamp for memorizing acupuncture
anesthesia
Issued on April 9th, 1976, collected
by Prof. ZHOU Jian-yang

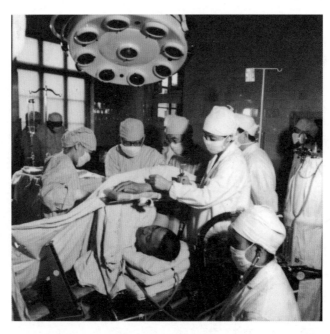

◇胸外科专家辛育龄在针麻下施行肺切除手术

北京结核病研究所,摄于 1979 年 6 月

Prof. XIN Yu-ling, a specialist of the chest surgery was performing a
pneumonoresection operation under acupuncture anesthesia
Taken in the Beijing Institute of Tuberculosis in June of 1979

# 75

## 尼克松访华掀起美国"针灸热"

President Nixon's visit to China set off an "acupuncture fever" in the U.S.

1972 年 2 月 21—28 日,美国总统尼克松应邀访华。24 日上午,美国国防部长黑格将军率领尼克松访华团随团官员和美国新闻媒体(尼克松和基辛格未到)共 30 余人,在北京医科大学第三附属医院观看了由辛育龄教授主刀、在针刺麻醉下施行"右肺上叶切除术"的全过程。手术后,手术医师与访问团座谈,答复美方提出的有关针麻镇痛原理和操作技术等问题。代表团返美后,纷纷宣传"针刺麻醉"的神奇,再一次引起美国民众兴趣,引发了美国以及世界范围内的针灸热潮。此次针刺麻醉手术,在开辟针灸走向美国的道路上起到了开创性作用。

From Febrary 21th to 28th, 1972, President Nixon was invited to visit China. In the morning of February 24th, more than 30 members of Nixon's China-visiting group led by General Alexander Meigs Haig, the Minister of Defense (without Nixon and Alfred Kissinger) observed the whole process of the "right-superior pulmonary loectomy" under acupuncture anesthesia. This operation was performed by Prof. XIN Yu-ling in the 3rd Affiliated Hospital of Beijing Medical University. After the operation, American visitors asked many questions related with the underlying mechanisms of acupuncture anesthesia, and its manipulation techniques. After the delegation returned home, American media publicized the mysterious acupuncture anesthesia in succession, arousing American people's great interest and initiating an upsurge of acupuncture research and clinical application in the U.S. and the world. This acupuncture anesthesia operation has a groundbreaking role in opening up acupuncture medicine to the U.S.

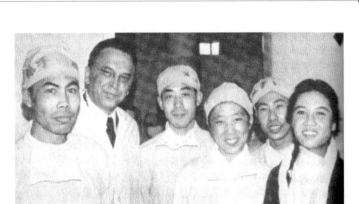

◇尼克松的私人医生塔卡（左2）在北京同针刺麻醉手术小组合影

引自《美国针灸热传奇》（李永明编著，人民卫生出版社，2011年）

Group photo of Dr. Walter Tkach (the 2$^{nd}$ one on the left, Nixon's private doctor) and acupuncture anesthesia group in Beijing.

Cited from book *Meiguo Zhenjiure Chuanqi* (《美国针灸热传奇》*Acupuncture Journey to America*), written by Dr. LI Yong-ming, published by People's Medical Publishing House in 2011

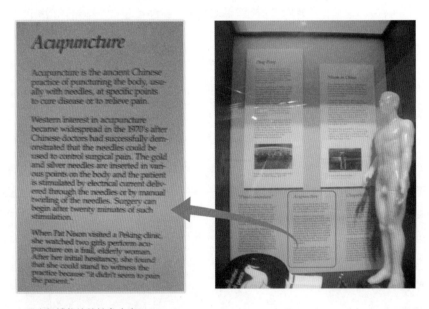

◇尼克松博物馆的针灸内容

摄于美国南加州尼克松博物馆

Acupuncture contents in the Nixon's Museum

Taken in the Nixon's Museum in South California of USA

尼克松访华掀起美国"针灸热"
President Nixon's visit to China set off an "acupuncture fever" in the U.S.

 ## 美国著名专栏作家接受针灸治疗

1971 年,为打破中美之间的外交坚冰,中国开展了以乒乓外交为代表的一系列外交活动,邀请美国著名专栏作家詹姆斯·赖斯顿(James Reston)访华就是其中之一。赖斯顿访华期间突患急性阑尾炎,于 1971 年 7 月 17—28 日,在北京的反帝医院(现北京协和医院)住院,接受阑尾切除术治疗,术中使用常规药物麻醉。

术后第 2 天,由于出现术后腹胀,赖斯顿接受了针刺和灸法的治疗,效果良好。1971 年 7 月 26 日,赖斯顿在美国《纽约时报》头版一角转第 6 版(几乎整版)发表了题为"现在让我告诉你们我在北京的阑尾切除手术"(Now, Let Me Tell You About My Appendectomy in Peking)的报道。赖斯顿痊愈之后,在上海观看了针刺麻醉手术,自此,美国媒体对中国针灸术的兴趣大增,为 1972 年尼克松访华后掀起的针灸热潮拉开了序幕。

## American famous columnist receiving acupuncture treatment

In 1971, in order to break the diplomatic ice between China and the United States, China launched a series of diplomatic activities represented by ping-pong (table tennis) diplomacy, among which James Reston, a famous American columnist, was invited to visit China. During his visit, James Reston suffered from acute appendicitis. He was hospitalized in Beijing's Anti-imperialist Hospital (now Peking Union Medical College Hospital) from July 17th to 28th, 1971, where he received an operation of appendectomy under routine anesthesia procedure.

On the second day after surgery, due to postoperative abdominal distention, James Reston received an acupuncture and moxibustion treatment with good effect. On July 26th, 1971, in *The New York Times*, Reston published a report entitled "Now, Let Me Tell You About My Appendectomy in Peking" in the 6th page (almost full page) with the title in the front page. After his recovery, he went to watch an operation with acupuncture anesthesia in Shanghai. Since then, American media showed great interest in Chinese acupuncture. The event raised an upsurge of Chinese acupuncture and moxibustion after Nixon's visit to China in 1972.

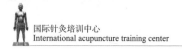
# 76

# 国际针灸培训中心
## International acupuncture training center

　　20 世纪 70 年代,随着针灸国际传播和交流的进一步发展,世界各国针灸爱好者学习针灸的愿望日益增长,为了适应需求,国内一些中医院校、针灸研究机构等陆续举办外国医师针灸学习班,接收外国学员学习针灸,为世界各地培养出一批针灸专业人才。

　　1975 年,受联合国世界卫生组织之委托,我国政府先后在中国中医研究院、上海中医学院、南京中医学院开办国际针灸班,向全世界招收学员。1983 年这 3 个国际针灸班分别更名为中国北京、上海、南京国际针灸培训中心,至今已为世界上 140 多个国家和地区培养了大量针灸人才。

In 1970s, along with the rapid development of propagation and international exchange of acupuncture and moxibustion, the acupuncture enthusiasts' aspiration for learning acupuncture and moxibustion gets increasing day by day. In order to adapt to the international requirements, some domestic colleges of TCM, research institutes of acupuncture-moxibustion, etc. have been holding batches of training classes in succession for foreign practitioners and have cultivated a large body of professionals for many regions of the world.

In 1975, entrusted by the World Health Organization (WHO), Chinese government opened three international acupuncture training classes in China Academy of Traditional Chinese Medicine (Beijing), Shanghai College of TCM and Nanjing College of TCM and recruited students from all over the world. In 1983, the three international acupuncture training classes were renamed as China Beijing International Acupuncture Training Center (CBITAC), Shanghai International Acupuncture Training Center and Nanjing International Acupuncture Training Center, and have cultivated a large body of acupuncture professionals for more than 140 countries and regions.

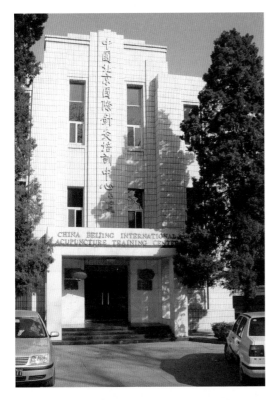

◇北京国际针灸培训中心原貌（1975—2010 年）

**Original appearance of Beijing International Acupuncture Training Center (1975–2010)**

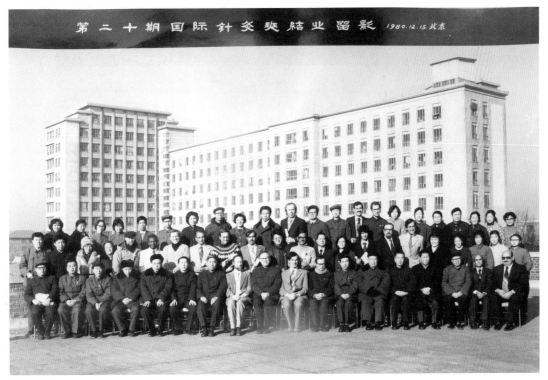

◇第 20 期北京国际针灸班结业留影（1980 年 12 月）

Group photo for the graduation ceremony of the 20th International Acupuncture Training Course, Beijing (December, 1980)

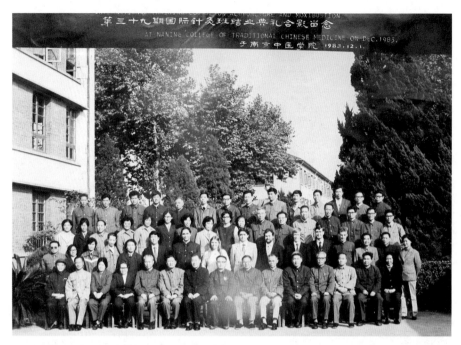

◇第 39 期南京国际针灸班结业典礼合影（1983 年 12 月）

Group photo for the graduation ceremony of the 39th International Acupuncture Training Course, Nanjing (December, 1983)

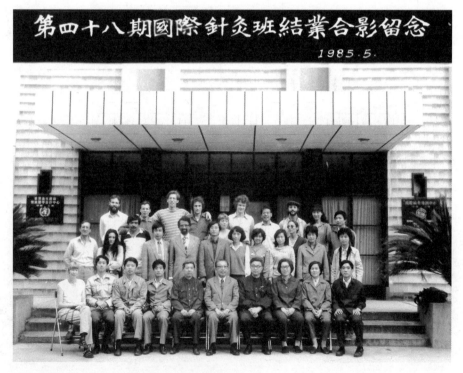

◇第 48 期上海国际针灸班结业合影（1985 年 5 月）

Group photo for the graduation ceremony of the 48th International Acupuncture Training Course, Shanghai (May, 1985)

# 77

## 针灸学术团体
### Academic societies of acupuncture and moxibustion

针灸学术团体,主要包括中国针灸学会和世界针灸学会联合会。

中国针灸学会于 1979 年 5 月 16 日成立,当时为中华全国中医学会的二级学会,1985 年 3 月 5 日升为国家一级学会。中国针灸学会按不同学科和专业,设立专业委员会(分会)和工作委员会。现设有临床、针法灸法、实验针灸、针刺麻醉、经络、腧穴、耳穴诊治、针灸文献等 28 个二级专业委员会(分会)以及标准化、学科与学术等 6 个工作委员会。

为促进世界针灸界之间的了解与合作,加强国际间的学术交流,1987 年 11 月 22 日,世界针灸学会联合会(WFAS)在北京成立。作为总部设在中国的非政府性针灸团体国际联合组织,目前已拥有团体会员 208 个,代表着 60 个国家和地区 30 余万名针灸工作者。世界针灸学会联合会的成立,标志着针灸国际交流发展到一个新阶段,将为人类健康做出更大的贡献。

The academic societies of acupuncture and moxibustion mainly include China Association of Acupuncture and Moxibustion (CAAM) and the World Federation of Acupuncture-moxibustion Societies (WFAS).

The CAAM, established on May 16th, 1979, was a second-order society of Chinese national society of TCM at the beginning, and became the first-order national society on March 5th, 1985. In the light of the subject and specialty, CAAM set up 28 speciality committees (second-order branch societies) as Clinic Branch, Needling and Moxibustion

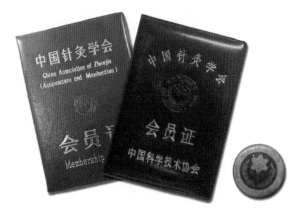

◇中国针灸学会会员证及徽标

Member card and logo of CAAM

Technique Branch, Experimental Acupuncture and Moxibustion Branch, Acupuncture Anesthesia Branch, Meridian-collateral Branch, Acupoint Branch, Otopoint Diagnosis-treatment Branch, Acupuncture-moxibustion Literature Branch, etc. as well as other 6 working committees as the Standardization Committee, Scientific Committee, Academic Committee, etc.

In order to facilitate the mutual understanding and co-operation in the acupuncture and moxibustion community, and to further strengthen international academic exchanges, the WFAS was established in Beijing on November 22$^{nd}$, 1987. It is a non-governmental international affiliation organization, with its headquarter founded in China. At the present, it has 208 group members and represents more than 300,000 of acupuncturists from 60 countries and regions. The foundation of WAFS indicates a new stage of the development of the international exchange for acupuncture and moxibustion, and will make a greater contribution to the health of the mankind.

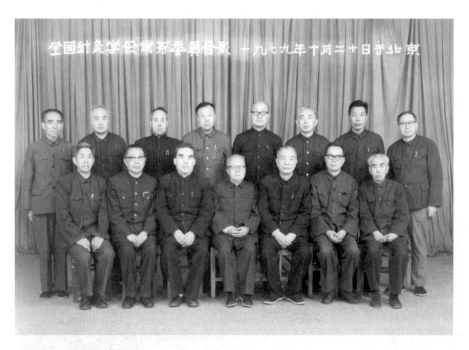

◇首届针灸学会常务委员合影

Group photo of the standing committee members of the first session of CAAM

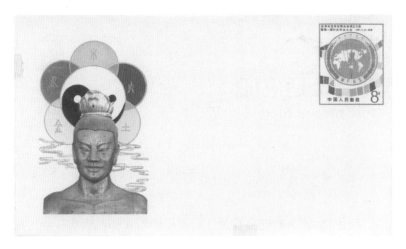

◇世界针灸学会联合会成立大会纪念邮资封

　1987 年 11 月发行,周建杨教授藏

Postage envelope for commemoration of WFAS

Issued in November of 1987, reserved by Prof. ZHOU Jian-yang

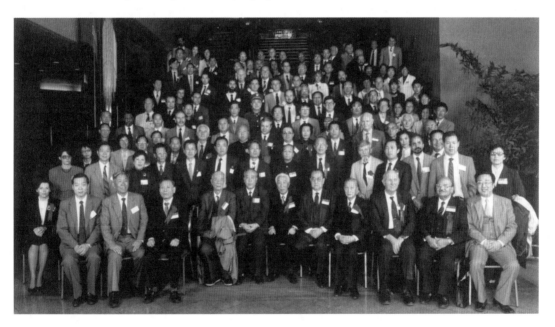

◇世界针灸学会联合会第一届会员大会代表合影( 1987 年 11 月 22 日 )

Group photo of member representatives of the 1st session of WFAS (November 22nd, 1987)

# 78

# 世界卫生组织推荐针灸适应证
## Indications for acupuncture recommended by WHO

　　随着针灸在世界范围内广泛传播,针灸的安全性及针灸到底能治疗哪些疾病一直困扰着使用者。世界卫生组织(WHO)自1980年始,数次公布针灸治疗的优势病种,鼓励全球患者选择针灸疗法。1979年,WHO在北京召开了地区间针灸、针麻学术会议,首次推荐43种针灸适应证,并于1980年以针灸专刊形式将其公布于《世界卫生》。1996年,WHO在意大利米兰召开会议,提出64种针灸适应证,并依据研究情况将其分为3类。2002年,WHO在《针灸临床研究报告的回顾与分析》中详细分析了针灸治疗病证的范围及疗效,根据研究进展将目前临床研究文献涉及的107种病证分为4类。

　　Along with the development of acupuncture and moxibustion in the world, its effectiveness, safety and indications became a main concern for users. Since 1980 WHO has issued for several times the recommended indications of acupuncture therapy, encouraging the global patients who seek complimentary and alternative therapies to chose this therapy. In 1979, WHO held regional academic congress on acupuncture and acupuncture anesthesia in Beijing, and for the first time issued 43 recommended indications for acupuncture and consequently published that on Acupuncture Special Issue of *World Health* in 1980. In 1996, WHO held a meeting in Milan of Italy to propose 64 indications for acupuncture which were classified into three categories accordingly. In 2002, WHO issued a report titled *Acupuncture: Review and Analysis of Reports on Controlled Clinical Trial* covering 107 illnesses or disorders of 4 categories, in which a detailed analysis on the range and effectiveness of diseases, symptoms or conditions for acupuncture therapy was made.

DOI:10.13424/j.cnki.jsctcm.1980.04.010

注为"气血之不能疏通者，宜按跷导引"。它可以防病强身益寿，达到为人民多作贡献的目的。

2、适应外界环境：通过身体的锻炼能适应外界气候的变化，避免外邪侵袭躯体，酿成疾病，所谓《素问•上古天真论曰》："虚邪贼风，避之有时"，《灵枢•本藏篇》云："寒温和，则六腑化谷，风痹不作，经脉通行，肢节得安"。《素问•生气通天论》云："清静，则肉腠闭拒，虽有大风苛毒，弗之能害"。尤其在强调作各种锻炼身体之前后，忌风着水受寒，以防气血受损。

3、劳逸结合：对于脑力劳动者，可以适当结合些肢体活动的锻炼，以作到有劳有逸，劳逸结合，《素问•宣明五气篇》云："久视伤血，久卧伤气，久坐伤肉，久立伤骨，久行伤筋"。说明机体在活动中，能正确运用，才能永保气血筋骨

正常，方不致发生疾病，正如汉、华佗说："流水不腐"的真意即在于此。

4、注意饮食：饮食对人体健康极为密切，如偏食或过食，又直接危害或影响身体的健康，正如《素问•上古天真论》曰："以酒为浆，以妄为常"等不正常的生活习惯，会严重损害人体健康，所以《素问•上古天真论》曰："饮食有节，起居有常"。可以永保气血筋骨的健壮。

5、加强安全教育：使人们在日常劳动中，明确"生产要安全，安全为了更好生产"的道理，并要言必行，行必果，方可杜绝异外事故的发生，造成气血筋骨的损伤。

总之，从以上看来，祖国医学在保养气血筋骨方面，积累了许多丰富而行之有效的理论和经验，其中许多方法，至今仍被广大群众行之有效，很值得发扬光大，造福于人民。

---

## 联合国世界卫生组织批准

# 用针刺疗法治疗四十三种疾病

根据1979年北京召开的世界卫生组织针灸针麻座谈会讨论的结果，提出针灸治疗的四十三种疾病名称如下：

上呼吸道疾病：急性鼻窦炎、急性鼻炎、感冒、急性扁桃体炎；

呼吸系统疾病：急性支气管炎、支气管哮喘（对儿童及无合并症者最有效）；

眼科疾病：急性结膜炎、中心性视网膜炎、近视（儿童）、白内障（无合并症者）；

口腔疾病：牙痛、拔牙后疼痛、牙龈炎、急或慢性咽炎；

胃肠疾病：食管贲门痉挛、呃逆、胃

下垂、急或慢性胃炎、胃酸过多、慢性十二指肠溃疡（缓解疼痛）、急性十二指肠溃疡（无合并症者）、急或慢性结肠炎、急性菌痢、便秘、腹泻、麻痹性肠梗阻；

神经和肌肉骨骼疾病：头痛、偏头痛、三叉神经痛、面瘫（早期，即3～6个月内）、中风后发生的不完全性瘫痪、外周性神经疾患、脊髓灰质炎后遗症（早期，6个月内）、美尼尔氏症、神经性膀胱功能障碍、夜尿症、肋间神经痛、颈臂综合症、"肩凝"、"网球肘"、坐骨神经痛、腰痛、骨关节炎。

（李焕斌整理）

—23—

◇世界卫生组织推荐的43种针灸适应证

引自《陕西中医学院学报》，1980年

43 indications of acupuncture recommended by WHO
Cited from the *Journal of Shaanxi College of Traditional Chinese Medicine* (1980)

伤及自由基损伤密切相关。本实验中，当我们给予外源性MT阻断剂或MAPK阻滞剂后，大鼠神经行为学评分出现显著减弱的趋势，电针抗氧应激的效应也被部分地阻断。由此我们推论：电针抗氧化效应与松果体素（MT）相关；电针抗氧化效应信号的一部分很可能通过MAPK信号途径的转导。另外，当用电针、MT、电针加MT治疗后，促凋亡基因Bax蛋白表达及Bax/Bcl-2同步有显著性意义地降低，抑凋亡基因Bcl-2蛋白的表达同步显著地提高，EA＋MT组表现得更明显。因此可以认为：在电针保护脑血性神经元及抗氧应激过程中，松果体素确实参与了抗氧应激、调节自由基损伤的整体效应。松果体激素MT是迄今为止发现的最强的内源性自由基清除剂，其基本功能是参与了机体的抗氧化系统，防止机体细胞过氧化损伤。MT抗氧化作用强度及清除羟自由基的能力是谷胱甘肽的4倍，甘露醇的10倍，Vit E的2倍；预防辐射自由基损伤是二甲亚砜的500倍；它可在某些过氧化氢酶缺乏或活性部位解除$H_2O_2$毒性，并与过氧化氢酶，谷胱甘肽氧化酶协同，以使细胞体内$H_2O_2$保持稳定。我们认为MT可能是电针抗氧化效应中十分重要的神经激素调质之一。

## 参考文献

1 Reiter R J, Tan D X, Qi W B. Suppression of oxygen toxicity by melatonin. Zhongguo Yao Li Xue Bao (Acta Pharmacol Sinica, Chin), 1998, 19(6): 575－581.

2 Li Z R, Sheng C R. Clinical study on acupuncture treatment of stroke and its mechanisms. Folia Sinotherapeutika (Belgium), 1992, 11(1): 18－22.

3 李忠仁，沈梅红，穆艳云. 针刺加当归芍药散治疗阿尔采默氏症的机理研究. 中华实用医药杂志, 2005, 5(10): 937－940.

Li Z R, Shen M H, Mu Y Y. Study on mechanisms underlying the treatment of Alzheimer's disease by acupuncture combined with Danggui Shaoyao San. Zhonghua Shi Yong Yi Yao Za Zhi (J Chin Pract Med, Chin), 2005, 5(10): 937－940.

4 李忠仁，崔　龙. TC指数在改良LONGA线栓法局灶性脑缺血/再灌注动物模型制备中的应用. 中国中西医结合杂志, 2006, 26(增刊): 18－20.

Li Z R, Cui L. Application of TC index location on LONGA's animal model of regional experimental cerebral ischemia and reperfusion. Zhongguo Zhong Xi Yi Jie He Za Zhi (Chin J Integr Trad West Med, Chin), 2006, 26(suppl): 18－20.

5 Kuluz J W, Prado R J, Dietrich W D, et al. The effect of nitric oxide-synthase inhibition on infarct volume after reversible focal cerebral ischemia in conscious rat. Stroke, 1993, 24(12): 2023－2029.

6 Garcia J H, Wagner S, Liu K F, et al. Neurological deficit and extent of neuronal necrosis attributable to middle cerebral artery occlusion in rat. Stroke, 1995, 26(4): 627－635.

7 李忠仁. 实验针灸学. 北京：中国中医药出版社, 2版, 2007: 255－257.

Li Z R. Experimental Acupuncturology (Chin). Beijing: China Press of Traditional Chinese Medicine, Second edition, 2007: 255－257.

8 Gu Z, Jiang Q, Zhang G, et al. Diphosphorylation of extracellular signal-regulated kinases and c-Jun N-terminal protein kinases in brain ischemic tolerance in rat. Brain Res, 2000, 860(1/2): 157－160.

（收稿日期：2007-10-26　修回日期：2008-03-10）

---

### 世界卫生组织认可的 64 种针灸适应证

为适应针灸临床治疗和研究发展需要, 1996 年 11 月召开了世界卫生组织意大利米兰会议, 提出 64 种针灸适应证, 并作如下论述:

(1) 采用类似针灸法或传统疗法随机对照试验过的针灸适应证有: 戒酒、变应性鼻炎(花粉症)、竞技综合症、面瘫、胆绞痛、支气管哮喘、心神经官能症、颈椎病、运动系统慢性疼痛(颈、肩、脊柱、膝等)、抑郁、戒毒、痛经、头痛、偏瘫或其它脑病后遗症、带状疱疹、高血压、原发性低血压、阳痿、引产、失眠、白细胞减少、腰痛、偏头痛、妊娠反应、恶心呕吐、肩周炎(冻结肩)、手术后疼痛、经前期紧张症、神经根疼痛综合症、肾绞痛、类风湿性关节炎、扭伤和劳损、下颌关节功能紊乱、紧张性头痛、戒烟、三叉神经痛、泌尿道结石。

(2) 有足够数量的病人为样本但无随机性对照试验的针灸适应证有: 急性扁桃体炎和急性咽喉炎、背痛、胆道蛔虫症、慢性咽炎、胎位不正、小儿遗尿、网球肘、胆结石、肠道激惹综合症、梅尼埃病、肌筋膜炎、儿童近视、单纯性肥胖、扁桃体切除术后疼痛、精神分裂症、坐骨神经痛。

(3) 有反复的临床报道, 效果较快或有一些试验依据的针灸适应证有: 便秘、缺乳、泄泻、女性不孕、胃下垂、呃逆、尿失禁、男性不育(精子缺乏、精子活动力缺乏)、无痛分娩、尿潴留、鼻窦炎。

◇世界卫生组织认可的 64 种针灸适应证

引自《针刺研究》杂志, 2008 年

64 indications of acupuncture approved by WHO

Cited from the journal *Acupuncture Research* (2008)

# 79

## 安徽省针灸医院
Anhui Hospital of Acupuncture and Moxibustion

1984 年,全国首家以针灸命名的专科医院——安徽中医学院附属针灸医院经省政府批准成立,其与安徽中医学院针灸经络研究所和安徽中医学院针灸系三位一体,医疗、教学、科研相互结合、优势互补。1985 年 2 月 4 日,安徽中医学院附属针灸医院在合肥市六安路原安徽中医学院第二门诊部的基础上正式挂牌开诊。2005 年被评为三级甲等中医专科医院。医院名称现为:安徽中医药大学第二附属医院、安徽省针灸医院。当前国内有针灸专科医院多家,其中较知名的还有山西省针灸医院、中国中医科学院针灸医院(其前身是 1951 年卫生部针灸疗法实验所门诊部)等。

In 1984, the first specialized acupuncture hospital, the Affiliated Hospital of Acupuncture and Moxibustion of Anhui College of TCM (current Anhui University of TCM) was established with the governmental approval. Thus, the affiliated hospital, Research Institute of Acupuncture-moxibustion and Meridians, and the Department of Acupuncture and Moxibustion (current the College of Acupuncture and Moxibustion) of Anhui University of TCM are trinity and complimentary to each other in medical treatment, education and scientific research. On February 4th 1985, the Affiliated Hospital of Anhui College of TCM was officially opened to public with its address on Liu-an Road of Hefei City where the 2nd Outpatient Department of Anhui College of TCM was located. In 2005, the Affiliated Hospital was awarded grade-3 specialized hospital of TCM, and currently renamed as the 2nd Affiliated Hospital and Anhui Provincial Hospital of Acupuncture and Moxibustion, Anhui University of TCM. At present in China, there have been several well-known specialty hospitals of acupuncture and moxibustion such as the Hospital of Acupuncture and Moxibustion of Shanxi Province, the Hospital of Acupuncture and Moxibustion of CACMS (its predecessor is the clinic of EIAMT subordinating to the Health Ministry founded in 1951), etc.

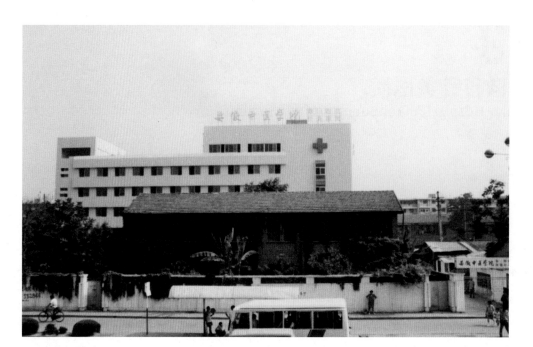

◇安徽省针灸医院外景

　摄于 1995 年

Outdoor scene of the Hospital of Acupuncture and Moxibustion of Anhui Province
Photographed in 1995

# 北京针灸学院
## Beijing College of Acupuncture and Moxibustion

为提高针灸学术水平,促进针灸事业发展和国际交流,也为了确保我国在中医学领域的优势,经国家计划委员会和教育部批准,1984年2月开始筹建北京针灸学院,1986年9月正式成立并招生,设置针灸学和骨伤科两个专业,学制均为五年,是我国第一所专门培养国内、国际高级针灸人才的高等学府,也是国内外针灸教育的重要基地之一。1987年该院更名为北京针灸骨伤学院,2001年7月1日合并到北京中医药大学。其实,早在1976年,就有过一个"南宁市七二一针灸大学",由著名针灸学家朱琏创办,至1980年共开办4届,培养针灸人才百余名,后停办。

In order to improve the academic level of acupuncture and moxibustion, promote the international exchange and to ensure the priority of China in the field of TCM, Beijing College of Acupuncture and Moxibustion started to be constructed in February 1984, approved by the State Planning Commission and Ministry of Education. In September of 1986, this college, the first high school for specially cultivating domestic and international high-ranking professionals of acupuncture and moxibustion was set up. It was composed of two majors, acupuncture-moxibustion and Osteo-traumatology for which the schooling system is 5 years, and is one of the important education bases for acupuncture and moxibustion. In 1987, Beijing College of Acupuncture and Moxibustion was renamed as Beijing College of Acupuncture and Moxibustion and Osteo-traumatology. On July 1st, 2001, this college was merged into Beijing University of \CM. In fact, early in 1976, there was already a university, named as 7 · 21 Acupuncture and Moxibustion University of Nanning City, established by ZHU Lian, the well-known acupuncturist. Before suspension, the university had fostered 4 sessions of graduates with over one hundred talents successfully.

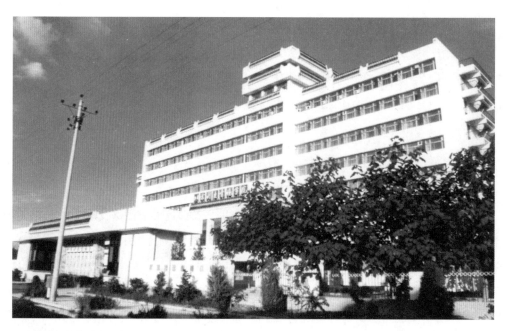

◇北京针灸骨伤学院原貌

The original appearance of Beijing College of Acupuncture and Moxibustion and Osteo-traumatology

# 81

## 针灸国家标准
State Standard of acupuncture and moxibustion of the People's Republic of China

　　20 世纪中期之前，在针灸发展史上虽无"标准"之名，早已有标准之实，如《灵枢·九针十二原》可谓是当时针具标准，《黄帝明堂经》总结了汉代之前的腧穴定位与主治，宋代王惟一奉敕编撰《铜人腧穴针灸图经》，铸造了针灸铜人以规范针灸教学与考试。这些可谓是针灸标准的肇始。

　　现代意义上的针灸国家标准化，始于 20 世纪 80 年代。第一部针灸国家标准是 1980 年由中国国家技术监督局发布的《针灸针》（GB 2024—80），后经 4 次修订为《针灸针》（GB 2024—2016）。20 世纪 90 年代，颁布了《经穴部位》（GB 12346—90）、《耳穴名称和部位》（GB/T 13734—92）。2000 年以来，陆续发布了 30 余项国家标准。

By the middle of the 20<sup>th</sup> century, the "standard" of acupuncture and moxibustion had already existed although no similar name was given. For example, the standardization-like words of acupuncture needles were mentioned in book *Lingshu: Jiuzhen Shier Yuan*, possibly being the ancient standards of acupuncture needles. In book *Huangdi Mingtang Jing*, the locations and indications of acupoints summarized before the Western Han Dynasty were recorded. And in the Song Dynasty, WANG Wei-yi was ordered to edit *Tongren Shuxue Zhenjiu Tujing* by the emperor and to cast bronze acupuncture figure for standardizing teaching and examination. All of those could be considered as the beginning of acupuncture standardization.

In the modern sense, the standardization of acupuncture and moxibustion began in 1980s. The first state standard of acupuncture-moxibustion is *Acupuncture Needle* (GB 2024–80) issued in 1980 by the State Administration of Technical Supervision of China, which was revised for four times as *Acupuncture Needle* (GB 2024–2016). In 1990s, the *Location of Points* (GB 12346–90) and *The Nomenclature and Location of Auricular Points* (GB/T 13734–92) were issued. Since 2000, more than 30 related state standards have been released successively.

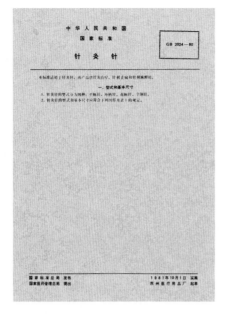

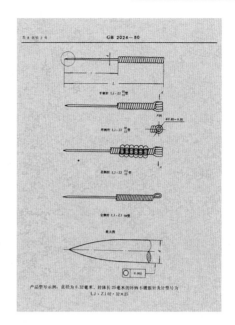

◇第一部针灸国家标准《针灸针》（GB 2024–80）

国家标准总局发布，1980 年

The first state standard of acupuncture and moxibustion: *Acupuncture Needle* (GB 2024–80)
Issued by the General Administration of National Standard of China in 1980

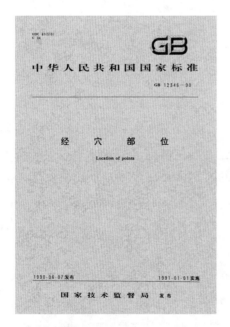

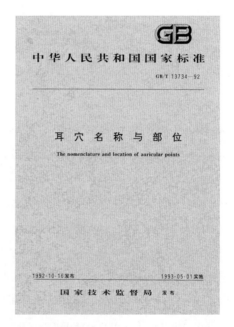

◇《经穴部位》（GB 12346–90）

国家技术监督局发布

*Location of Points* (GB 12346–90)
Issued by the State Administration of Technical
Supervision of China

◇《耳穴名称和部位》（GB/T 13734–92）

国家技术监督局发布

*The Nomenclature and Location of Auricular Points*
(GB/T 13734–92)
Issued by the State Administration of Technical
Supervision of China

# 82

## 针灸国际标准
## International standardization of acupuncture and moxibustion

    针灸国际标准化,始于 20 世纪 80 年代,最早的针灸国际标准是 1984 年世界卫生组织西太区出版的针灸命名标准(Standard Acupuncture Nomenclature)。1989 年,世界卫生组织总部召开国际标准针灸穴名科学组会议,审议和采纳了该西太区标准,于 1991 年发布修订版,包括十四经穴(361 个)的标准命名及穴名简释、经外奇穴(48 个)的标准命名、头皮针(14 个)的标准命名、耳穴(79 个)的标准命名、奇经八脉的标准命名及针灸基本术语的标准命名、针灸针的标准命名、针灸测量单位的标准命名。

    世界卫生组织先后颁布了"针灸临床研究方法指南"(1995),"针灸基础培训与安全规范"(1998)及"针灸经穴定位"(2008)。2009 年,国际标准化组织(International Organization for Standardization, ISO)成立中医技术委员会(ISO/TC249),目前已发布"一次性使用无菌针灸针""艾灸器""刮痧板"及"皮内针"4 个 ISO 针灸国际标准。这些标准对促进针灸的国际教学、科研、临床实践与信息的交流,起到了重要的作用。

    The international standardization of acupuncture and moxibustion started from 1980s. In 1984, the *Standard Acupuncture Nomenclature* issued by WHO Regional Office for the Western Pacific (WPRO) was the earliest publication. In 1989, WHO held a scientific group meeting at the headquarters to examine the Standard Acupuncture Point Locations proposed by WHO WPRO, adopted this standard and published the revised version in 1991. The revised version covers the standard nomenclature of classical acupuncture points of the 14 regular meridians (361 acupoints) with simple explanations of the points, the standard nomenclature of the extraordinary points (48 acupoints), the standard nomenclature of the scalp acupuncture (14 acupoints); the standard nomenclature of the auricular points (79 acupoints), the standard nomenclature of the eight extra meridians, the standard nomenclature of acupuncture basic terminology, the standard nomenclature of the acupuncture needle and the standard nomenclature of measurement unit.

    WHO successively issued *Guidelines on Clinical Research Methology in Acupuncture* (1995),

*Guidelines on Basic Training and Safety in Acupuncture* (1998) and *Standard of Acupuncture Point Locations* (2008). In 2009, the International Organization for Standardization (ISO) set up a Traditional Chinese Medicine Technology Committee (ISO/TC249). Till now, there have been four international acupuncture standards issued, namely "Sterile Acupuncture Needles for Single Use", "Moxibustion Device", "Scraping Device" and "Intradermal Needle". These standards may play an important role in promoting international education, scientific research, clinical practice and information exchange on acupuncture.

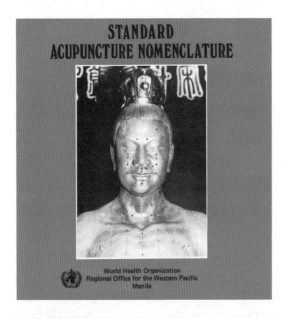

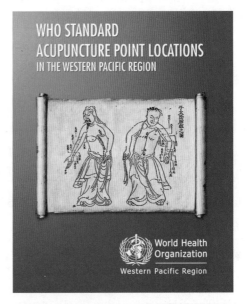

◇针灸命名标准

　　世界卫生组织西太区办公室发布, 1984 年

*Standard Acupuncture Nomenclature*
Issued by WHO Regional Office for the Western Pacific in 1984

◇针灸经穴定位标准

　　世界卫生组织西太区办公室发布, 2008 年

*WHO Standard Acupuncture Point Locations in the Western Pacific Region*
Issued by WHO Regional Office for the Western Pacific in 2008

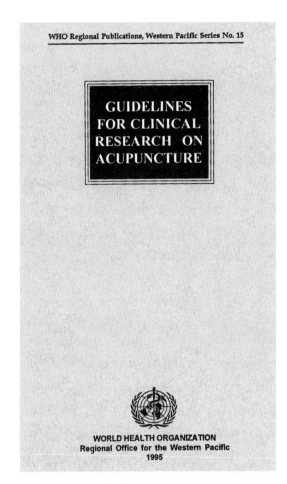

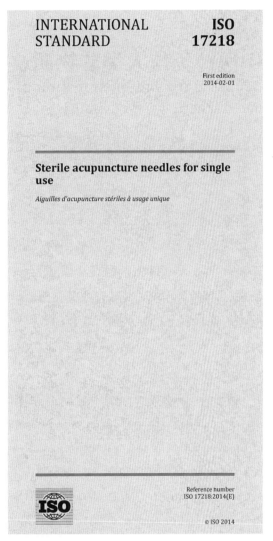

◇针灸临床研究方法指南

　　世界卫生组织西太区办公室发布，1995 年

*Guidelines for Clinical Research on Acupuncture*
Issued by WHO Regional Office for the Western Pacific in 1995

◇一次性使用无菌针灸针标准

　　国际标准化组织发布，2014 年

Standard of *Sterile Acupuncture Needles for Single Use*
Issued by International Organization for Standardization (ISO) in 2014

# 83

# 中医针灸与人类非物质文化遗产
## Acupuncture and moxibustion of TCM and intangible cultural heritage of humanity

中医针灸，是在中国独立起源、形成、发展起来的，历史悠久，具有鲜明的中国传统文化特质，数千来为中华民族的繁衍昌盛做出了贡献，是世界非物质文化遗产的一部分。2006年7月，国家中医药管理局成立了"中国传统医药申报世界文化遗产委员会"及其办公室，具体负责传统医药非物质文化遗产申报与保护工作。2010年11月16日由中国申报的"中医针灸"项目正式通过联合国教科文组织（UNESCO）保护非物质文化遗产政府间委员会第5次会议审议，被列入"人类非物质文化遗产代表作名录"。

Acupuncture and moxibustion of TCM originated and developed from China with long history and distinctive traditional Chinese culture feature. It has contributed a lot to the prosperity of Chinese nation in the past thousands of years, and is an integral part of the world intangible cultural heritage. In July 2006, the State Administration of TCM of the People's Republic of China set up "Committee for the Declaration of TCM as World Cultural Heritage" and its office for the declaration and protection of TCM as world intangible cultural heritage. On November 16th, 2010, China's "Acupuncture and Moxibustion of TCM" was officially approved to be included in the list of "Intangible Cultural Heritage of Humanity" by the 5th session of the United Nations Educational, Scientific and Cultural Organization (UNESCO) intergovernmental committee, for the safeguarding of the intangible cultural heritage.

# Convention for the Safeguarding of the Intangible Cultural Heritage

United Nations
Educational, Scientific and
Cultural Organization

Intangible
Cultural
Heritage

The Intergovernmental Committee for the Safeguarding of the Intangible Cultural Heritage has inscribed

*Acupuncture and moxibustion of traditional Chinese medicine*

on the Representative List of the Intangible Cultural Heritage of Humanity upon the proposal of China

*Inscription on this List contributes to ensuring better visibility of the intangible cultural heritage and awareness of its significance, and to encouraging dialogue which respects cultural diversity*

Date of inscription
*16 November 2010*

Director-General of UNESCO
*Irina Bokova*

◇ "中医针灸" 列入人类非物质文化遗产代表作名录证书（2010 年 11 月 16 日）

Certificate for "Acupuncture and Moxibustion of TCM" inscribed into the list of "Intangible Cultural Heritage of Humanity" (November 16th, 2010)

# 84

## 习近平向世界卫生组织赠送"针灸铜人"

## President XI Jin-ping presented "acupuncture bronze statue" as a gift to WHO

2017 年 1 月 18 日,国家主席习近平在日内瓦访问世界卫生组织,并赠送"针灸铜人"雕塑。该具铜人以现存于中国国家博物馆的针灸铜人为原型,铜人高 1.8 米,全身标注 559 个穴位,其中 107 个穴位是一名二穴,共计 666 个针灸点。在设计制作上应用 3D 建模技术,工艺采用中国传统的青铜失蜡浇铸法,在文物原型的基础上,对人体结构、穴位、文字、纹饰、雕塑表面等进行优化设计,追求科学性与艺术性的相结合。

在铜人赠送仪式上,习主席致辞指出,我们要继承好、发展好、利用好传统医学,用开放包容的心态促进传统医学和现代医学更好融合。

On January 18th, 2017, Xi Jin-ping, the president of the People's Republic of China, visited WHO in Geneva and presented "acupuncture bronze statue" as a gift to WHO. This bronze statue is a replica of the acupuncture bronze statue preserved nowadays in the National Museum of China, being 1.8 meter in height and marked with 559 acupoints (including 107 points of bilateral sides, actually 666 in total). The statue was made by using 3D modeling technique, Chinese traditional bronze dewaxing casting technique, and mostly optimum design on the human structure, acupoints, characters, decoration, sculptural surface, etc., reflecting the scientific and artistic perfect combination.

During the presentation ceremony, President XI pointed out that we should make traditional medicine better inherited, well developed and properly utilized, and promote the integration of traditional medicine and modern medicine with an open and inclusive attitude.

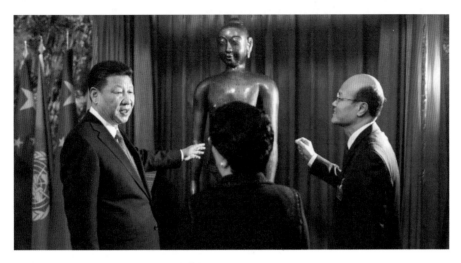

◇习近平主席向世界卫生组织赠送"针灸铜人"

引自世界卫生组织中国网站

President XI Jin-ping was presenting "acupuncture bronze statue" as a gift to WHO
Cited from the website of World Health Organization

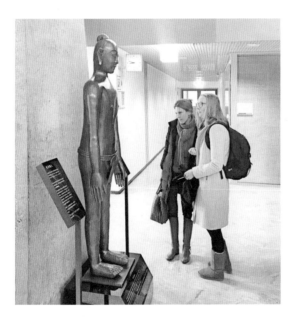

◇习主席赠送的"针灸铜人"摆放在世界卫生组织总部大厅

Acupuncture bronze statue presented by President XI in the hall of WHO